THE CEO MENU
FALL EDITION

JILL TREAT
MEAL PRO

A SIMPLE LIFE

TREAT YOURSELF SIMPLE

IS A HAPPY LIFE

BOOKS

The CEO Menu: Fall Edition
Author: Jill Treat

Published by Treat Yourself Simple Books
Marshall, Michigan, USA

www.facebook.com/GetMoreProductivity

Contact publisher for bulk orders and permission requests.

Cover and interior book design & formatting by **Leesa Ellis** of **3 ferns** » 3ferns.com
Self-publishing consultancy by **3 ferns** » 3ferns.com

Photography by Jill Treat

Printed in the United States of America.

ISBN (hardcover):   979-8-9912991-0-7
ISBN (paperback):   979-8-9912991-1-4

Also available for Kindle and other eBook devices

CONTENTS

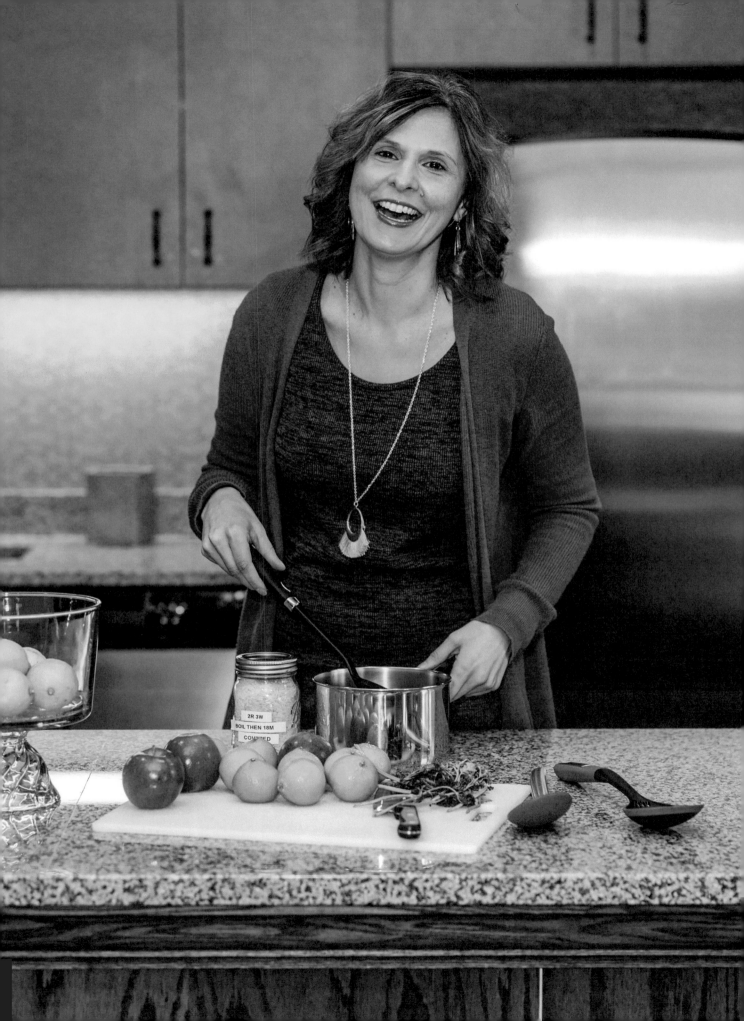

TO MY MOM

Your love, patience, and culinary wisdom
have not only shaped the outcome
of this book, but gave us the opportunity
to go through this journey together.

Thank you for coming to my place
to help do whatever was needed,
from washing dishes to prepping the food
and making the notes. I don't know how
I would have done it without you.

Thank you for teaching me
that food is not just about nourishment,
but about connection, celebration, and family.
This book is for you, with all my love.

JILL

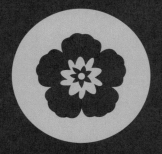

JILL TREAT
MEAL PRO

WELCOME TO THE FAMILY!

The purpose of this book is to help ease your mind by bringing clarity around the simple question: "What should I eat?" Not by simply answering this question, but by truly understanding it, so that the answer we provide actually aids you in attaining the highest level of achievement in your career.

The following menu plans have been put together not only to create balanced meals, but specifically to help you obtain the energy needed in order to fulfill your goals in each aspect of your life – professional and personal.

You will find weekly menus, recipe-specific grocery lists, and delicious easy recipes.

Remember, the recipes provided are designed as a flexible menu plan to fit your lifestyle.

So here's how this easy to use system works:

- ○ **Pick out 3–5 recipes.**
- ○ **Shop your kitchen for the ingredients needed.**
- ○ **Order or shop at the local market.**
- ○ **Make sure to get prepped ingredients if you don't have time or don't want to prep.**
- ○ **Chop/cut/dice ingredients.**
- ○ **Prepare ingredients per the Instructions.**
- ○ **Simply finish or heat the ingredients per Recipe.**
- ○ **Sides are recommended but can be switched out according to desired preference or availability.**

ENJOY!

Some nights, we just don't have as much time as we'd like, and that's when this book will come in handy as Plan B... to avoid the stress and scrambling as soon as it's time to eat.

Through having just a few of the suggested ingredients in your kitchen, quick and easy dinners will become your new normal, so you have more time (and energy) to focus on what's really important.

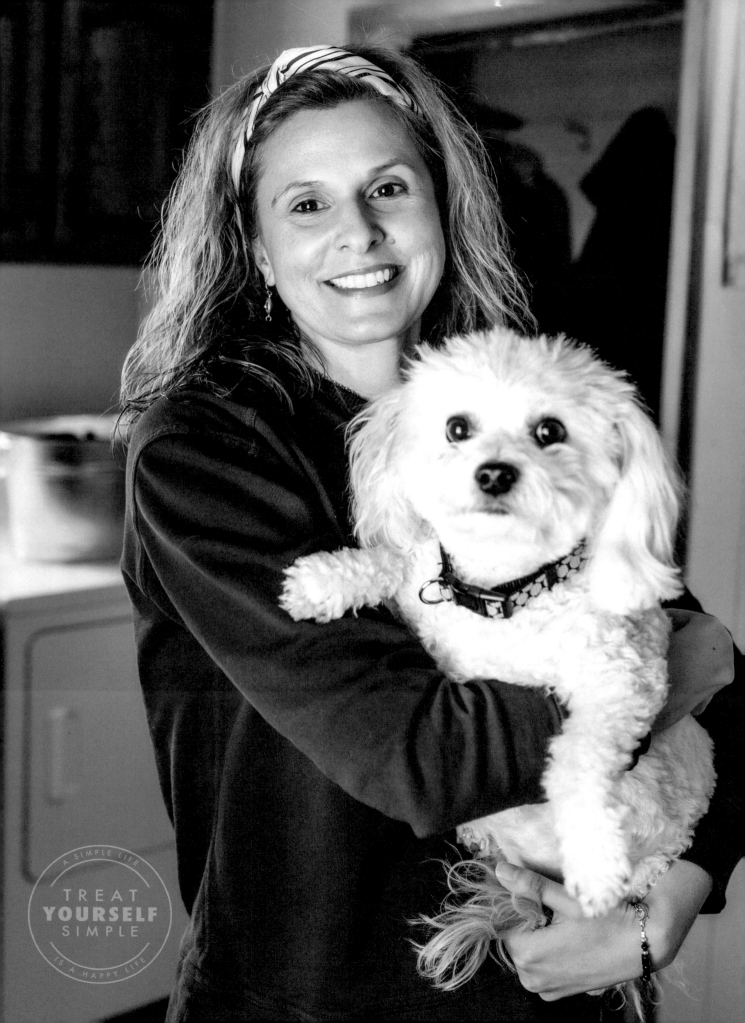

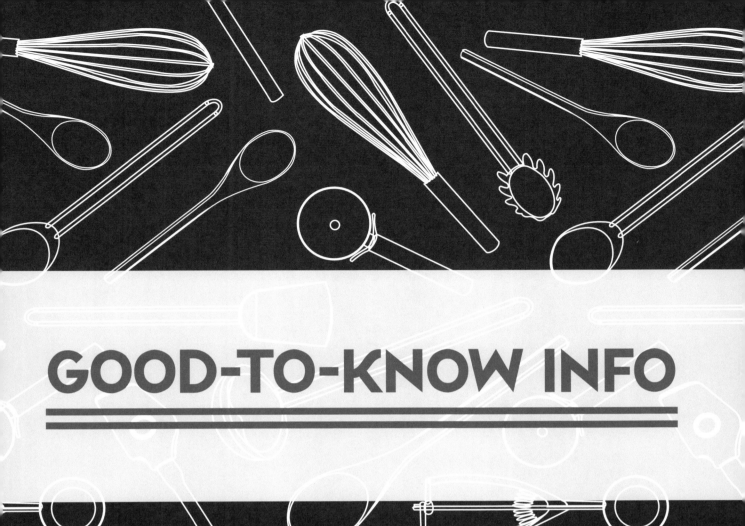

GOOD-TO-KNOW INFO

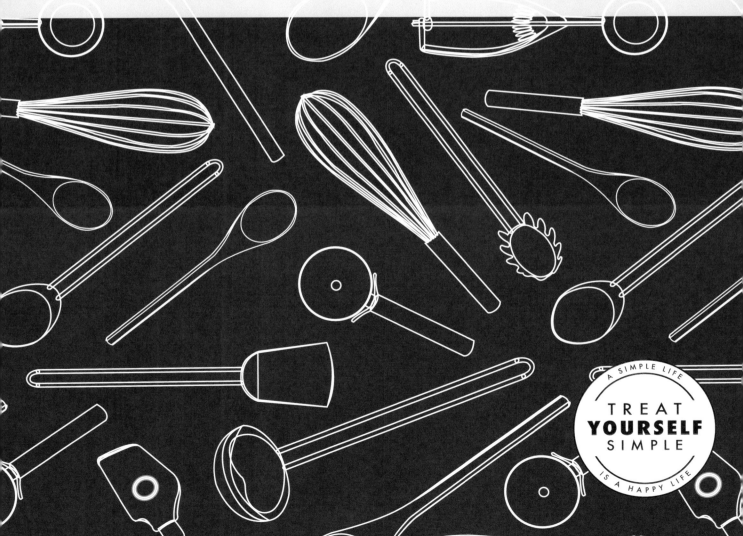

A SIMPLE LIFE
TREAT
YOURSELF
SIMPLE
IS A HAPPY LIFE

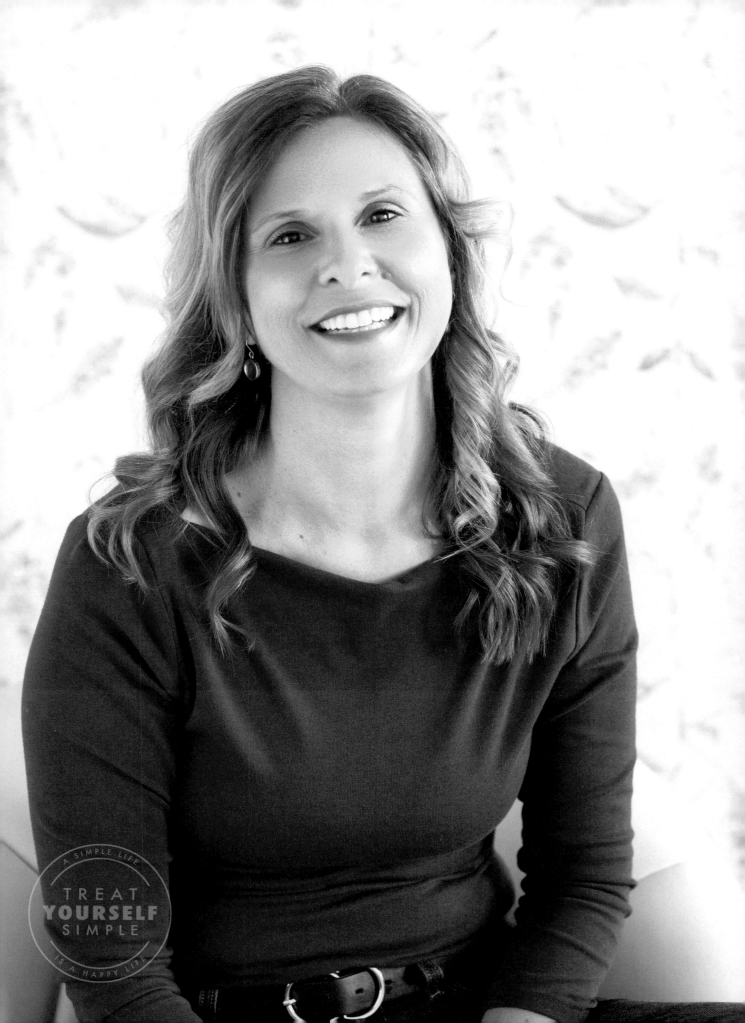

SIMPLE SUBSTITUTIONS

T
he purpose of this section is for you to be able to shop your kitchen, then order the groceries. We do not need a huge stockpile of food we are never going to eat. I suggest maybe having a few of the staples that I use every week on hand for easy meal prep. Plus you know what you like, there's no need to change.

PROTEIN SWAPS

Make protein substitutions according to preference and/or what you have on hand, adjusting cook times accordingly. For faster cooking time, adjust the size of the protein by cutting it into smaller pieces (or remove the meat from the bones) so it cooks faster; keep in mind, larger pieces will cook at a slower rate.

INGREDIENT	SUBSTITUTION
BEEF	
Ground Beef	Ground Chicken, Ground Pork, Ground Turkey
Sirloin Steak	New York Strip Steak, Ribeye
POULTRY	
Ground Chicken	Ground Pork, Ground Turkey
Chicken Breasts	Boneless skinless Chicken Thighs, Turkey Breasts, Extra-Lean Ground Turkey
PORK	
Ground Pork	Ground Beef, Ground Chicken, Ground Turkey
Pork Chops	Chicken, Pork Tenderloin, Pork Shoulder Steak, Tofu, Portobello Mushrooms
SEAFOOD	
Lean Fish	Bass, Catfish, Cod, Flounder, Halibut, Monkfish, Red Snapper, Skate, Sole, Tilapia
Fatty Fish	Char, Mahi-Mahi, Salmon, Swordfish, Tuna
Shrimp	King Oyster Mushrooms, Tofu, Chicken, Tilapia, Cod

HEALTHY COOKING OILS

Oils come in handy for making your own salad dressings, marinades, dips, and sauces. They are also great to use when grilling, baking or roasting foods. Oils coat pans to keep food from sticking. You can lightly drizzle on foods for flavor. And last but not least, you can season cast iron cookware.

Common "Better-for-You" Cooking Oils	Canola, Corn, Olive, Safflower, Sunflower, Vegetable
Speciality Oils	Avocado, Grapeseed, and Sesame

GARLIC

While it does flavor dishes, garlic is actually considered a "Root Vegetable".

FRESH GARLIC CLOVES	JARRED MINCED GARLIC	GARLIC POWDER
1	½ teaspoon	½ teaspoon

HERBS

INGREDIENT	SUBSTITUTION
Basil	Cilantro, Dill, Italian Seasoning, Oregano, Mint, Parsley
Cilantro	Basil, Parsley, Mint
Dill	Basil, Mint, Parsley
Mint	Basil, Cilantro, Dill, Parsley
Parsley	Basil, Chives, Cilantro, Dill, Italian Seasoning, Mint
Bay Leaves	Oregano, Rosemary, Sage, Thyme
Oregano	Bay Leaves, Italian Seasoning, Rosemary, Thyme, Sage
Rosemary	Bay Leaves, Oregano, Thyme, Sage
Sage	Bay Leaves, Oregano, Rosemary, Thyme
Thyme	Bay Leaves, Oregano, Rosemary, Sage

NOTES

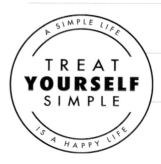

SPICES

INGREDIENT	SUBSTITUTION
Allspice	Combine Cinnamon, Cloves And Nutmeg, or use any one of the three
Chili Powder	Combine Paprika, Onion Powder, Garlic Powder, Cumin, Oregano And Cayenne Or Red-Pepper Flakes; Or Use Another Warm Spice, Such As Cayenne, Cloves, Cumin, Nutmeg Or Paprika
Cinnamon Blend	Allspice, Apple Pie Spice Blend, Cloves, Coriander, Nutmeg, Pumpkin Pie Spice
Cloves	Allspice, Cinnamon, Nutmeg, Black Pepper
Cumin	Chili Powder, Coriander, Curry Powder, Garlic Powder, Onion Powder, Turmeric
Curry Powder	Garlic Powder, Onion Powder, Turmeric
Garlic Powder	Curry Powder, Onion Powder, Turmeric
Ginger	Allspice, Cinnamon, Cloves, Coriander
Nutmeg	Allspice, Cinnamon, Cloves, Ground Ginger
Onion Powder	Curry Powder, Garlic Powder, Turmeric
Paprika	Cayenne, Chili Powder, Curry Powder, Black Pepper

NOTES

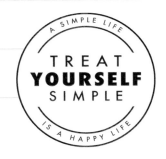

VEGETABLES

Substituting vegetables can be tricky, and depends largely on taste. But some can definitely step in for others: say Brussels sprouts for broccoli. Just bear in mind texture, moisture content and density.

COOK TIME	SUBSITITUTION
Quick-Cooking	Cabbage, Bok Choy, Broccoli, Broccolini, Brussels Sprouts, Cauliflower, Green Beans, Celery, Corn, Eggplant, Fennel, Mushrooms, Peas, Peppers, Zucchini
Slower-Cooking	Beet, Carrot, Parsnip, Potato, Sweet Potato, Turnip, Butternut Squash, Pumpkin

INGREDIENT	SUBSTITUTION
Onions	Leeks, Onions (Red, White or Yellow), Scallions, Shallots
Bell Peppers	Any color can be used in each recipe. Sometimes I just like my food to look a certain way.
Baby Spinach	Kale, Swiss Chard, Arugula, Romaine Lettuce, Collard Greens, Watercress, Cabbage, Microgreens
Arugula	Spinach, Basil, Romaine

DAIRY

Flavor and texture are important considerations when substituting dairy products.

INGREDIENT	SUBSTITUTION
Milk	Half & Half or Heavy Cream thinned with water, Evaporated Milk, Light Coconut Milk, Light Cream, Oat Milk, Nut Milk, Soy Milk
Half & Half	Thicken Milk (use any of above options) with a little cornstarch or flour (about 1 tablespoon per cup of liquid) or thin Heavy Cream with a splash of water,
Heavy Cream	For 1 cup Heavy Cream, use ¾ cup milk and ¼ cup melted butter, or thicken 1 cup milk with 1 to 2 tablespoons cornstarch or flour (whisk milk into cornstarch or flour little by little.) Coconut Milk, Coconut Cream (beware of increased sweetness), or Cream Cheese whisked with a little water also work.

CHEESES

Yes, you can interchange your cheeses in these recipes. Please note switches can alter the flavor of the recipe.

INGREDIENT	SUBSTITUTION
CHEDDAR	
Dairy	Gruyère, Gouda, Brie, Monterey Jack, Parmesan, Fontina, Havarti, Provolone, Swiss
Dairy-Free	Hummus, Dairy-Free Pesto, Brazil Nuts, Nutritional Yeast, Olives, Sun-Dried Tomatoes, Salt-Roasted Almonds, Sea Salt, Capers, Toasted Breadcrumbs
COLBY JACK	
Dairy	Monterey Jack, Mild or Medium Cheddar
Dairy-Free	Hummus, Dairy-Free Pesto, Brazil Nuts, Nutritional Yeast, Olives, Sun-Dried Tomatoes, Salt-Roasted Almonds, Sea Salt, Capers, Toasted Breadcrumbs
MEXICAN	
Dairy	Cotija, Feta, Parmesan
Dairy-Free	Brazil Nuts, Nutritional Yeast, Olives, Sun-Dried Tomatoes, Salt-Roasted Almonds, Sea Salt, Capers, Toasted Breadcrumbs
GOUDA	
Dairy	Cheddar, Provolone, Gruyère, Munster, Havarti
Dairy-Free	Hummus, Dairy-Free Pesto, Brazil Nuts, Nutritional Yeast, Olives, Sun-Dried Tomatoes, Salt-Roasted Almonds, Sea Salt, Capers, Toasted Breadcrumbs
GRUYÈRE	
Dairy	American Swiss, Mozzarella, Provolone, Parmesan, Feta, Goat Cheese
Dairy-Free	Hummus, Dairy-Free Pesto, Brazil Nuts, Nutritional Yeast, Olives, Sun-Dried Tomatoes, Salt-Roasted Almonds, Sea Salt, Capers, Toasted Breadcrumbs
MOZZARELLA	
Dairy	Gruyère, Cheddar, Swiss, Ricotta, Provolone, Fontina, Parmesan
Dairy-Free	Hummus, Dairy-Free Pesto, Brazil Nuts, Olives, Sun-Dried Tomatoes, Salt Roasted Almonds, Cashews, Sea Salt, Capers, Toasted Breadcrumbs

PARMESAN	
Dairy	Feta, Cheddar, Gruyère
Dairy-Free	Brazil Nuts, Nutritional Yeast, Olives, Sun-Dried Tomatoes, Salt-Roasted Almonds, Sea Salt, Capers, Toasted Breadcrumbs

FETA	
Dairy	Goat Cheese, Parmesan, Cottage Cheese
Dairy-Free	Olives, Sun-Dried Tomatoes, Salt-Roasted Almonds, Sea Salt, Capers, Hummus, Avocado

BLUE CHEESE	
Dairy	Goat Cheese. Cream Cheese, Feta, Cottage Cheese, Ricotta Cheese, Parmesan, Greek Yogurt
Dairy-Free	Roasted Nuts, Olives, Hummus, Avocado, Sun-Dried Tomatoes, Capers

NOTES

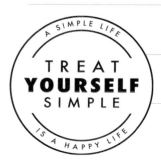

A SIMPLE LIFE
TREAT
YOURSELF
SIMPLE
IS A HAPPY LIFE

SEASONAL SIDES

Fall is a time to gather and harvest the fruits of our labor. This time of year I think of the Friday Night Football games, hay rides, bonfires, and some good produce. One thing when you work with Treat Yourself Simple is our promotion of **SEASONAL FRUITS & VEGGIES**.

Let's get real...

○ We want to save money on food costs.

○ We want to get the most nutritional value.

○ We want to be able to use our time wisely to stay focused on what you do best!

○ That's exactly why we focus on using/utilizing my favorite fall ingredients.

FRESH FRUIT
2 SERVINGS ~ NO COOK

FRUIT	COMPLEMENTARY INGREDIENT
2 Apples	4 T Nut Butter
2 Pears	2 oz Goat Cheese
2 Bananas	½ -1 T Cinnamon
2 C Pomegranate	2 t Honey and 1 C Yogurt

SPICED FRUIT
2 SERVINGS ~ OVEN

2–3 ⮞ Apples, Pears, medium

1 T ⮞ Butter or Coconut Oil

½ t ⮞ Cinnamon

○ Preheat the oven to 350° F.

○ Put the fruit in medium baking dish. Drizzle the melted butter or coconut oil over fruit. Sprinkle with cinnamon. Toss well to coat all pieces of fruit.

○ Bake in the preheated oven until the fruit pieces are soft, about 10-15 minutes. Stir once during the baking time. Enjoy!

ROASTED VEGETABLES

2 SERVINGS ~ OVEN

1–2 C ➤ Vegetables, fresh

1 T ➤ Olive Oil

○ Preheat the oven to 350° F.

○ Place vegetables on baking sheet

○ Drizzle olive oil over vegetables

○ Stir to coat vegetables

○ Bake in preheated oven for 20 minutes. Enjoy!

NOTE: *If frozen, prepare per instructions on the package.*

FRESH SALAD

2 SERVINGS ~ NO COOK

2 C ➤ Greens

○ In a large bowl, add one or a mixture of greens.

1 C ➤ Favorite Veggies or Fruits

○ Add a combination of fresh veggies such as: cucumbers, peppers, shredded carrots, tomatoes.

4 T ➤ Dressing

○ Drizzle with your favorite dressing. Season to taste with flaky sea salt, if desired.

NOTES

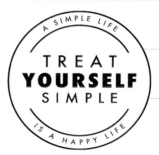

COLESLAW

2 SERVINGS ~ NO COOK

¼ C ⊱ Mayonnaise

½ T ⊱ Sugar, granulated

½ T ⊱ Apple Cider Vinegar, may substitute Distilled, White Wine, or Red Wine Vinegar

dash ⊱ Table Salt

dash ⊱ Black Pepper, ground

○ In a small dish, prepare the dressing by whisking above ingredients together.

1 C ⊱ Cabbage, green, shredded (can use pre-shredded cabbage)

⅓ C ⊱ Cabbage, purple, shredded (can use pre-shredded cabbage)

⅓ C ⊱ Carrots, peeled, shredded

○ In a large bowl, toss together the above ingredients.

○ Drizzle dressing over cabbage/carrot mixture and toss/stir until ingredients are thoroughly combined and all cabbage/carrots are coated with dressing. Taste-test and add more salt & pepper as needed.

○ Cover and refrigerate for at least 1 hour before serving (for best flavor).

SWEET POTATOES DISCS

2 SERVINGS ~ OVEN

2 ⊱ Sweet Potatoes, large, sliced ¼–⅓" thick, with skin

2–3 T ⊱ Olive Oil

○ Preheat the oven to 425º F.

○ Place sweet potato slices on baking sheet.

○ Brush olive oil over sweet potato slices; season with lemon pepper, flip and repeat on the other side.

○ Bake for 20 minutes. Use spatula to flip sweet potato slices.

○ Bake for an additional 20 minutes until both sides are browned and crisp.. Enjoy!

RICE
2 SERVINGS ~ STOVE

1 C ➤ Rice, Jasmine, Wild, or Brown

1¼ C ➤ Water

- ○ Let's make this easy. No rinsing required.

- ○ Place ingredients in saucepan and bring to a simmer on high heat.

- ○ Cover and turn to low heat for 12 minutes. Do not lift lid.

- ○ Stand 10 minutes to let the rice finish cooking.

- ○ Fluff with a fork. Serve warm.

    NOTE: *If not needed, cool, store in an airtight container/zip top bag in 2 serving portions. Refrigerate for up to 7 days. Freeze for up to 3 months .*

BLACK BEANS & RICE ~ ZATARAIN'S PACKAGE
4 SERVINGS

- ○ Prepare black beans and rice according to package instructions. Serve warm.

    NOTE: *If not needed, cool, store in an airtight container/zip top bag in 2 serving portions. Refrigerate for up to 7 days. Freeze for up to 3 months.*

QUINOA ~ SUCCESS
2 SERVINGS ~ STOVE

- ○ Follow directions on package. Serve warm.

    NOTE: *Cool, store in an airtight container/zip top bag in 2 serving portions. Refrigerate for up to 7 days.*

REFRIED BEANS ~ USE CHOICE OF CANNED

- ○ Heat skillet over medium heat, drizzle with oil. Add beans and heat for 3–5 minutes or desired temperature is reached. Serve warm.

MAKE AHEAD & PREP RECIPES

MINCED GARLIC

GARLIC CLOVES

○ Line up your peeled garlic cloves.

○ Slice off and discard any dry-looking ends.

○ Set the top of your knife on your cutting board. Place your non-dominant hand on top of the knife to steady it. Start chopping the garlic by fanning your knife back and forth in a rocking motion. Keep the tip of your knife in contact with the board while you fan. Keep at it until you have tiny pieces of minced garlic.

NOTE: *Store in the refrigerator for 7 days in an airtight container. Freeze up to 6 months in an airtight container.*

SHRED CHEESE

BLOCK CHEESE

○ Shred desired amount with a grater.

NOTE: *Store in refrigerator for 7 days in an airtight container. Freeze for up to 6 months.*

TACO SEASONING

APPROXIMATELY 8 SERVINGS

1 T ⌐ Chili Powder
½ T ⌐ Cumin
½ t ⌐ Onion Powder
¼ t ⌐ Garlic Powder
¼ t ⌐ Red Pepper Flakes
½ t ⌐ Oregano, dried
½ t ⌐ Kosher Salt
1 t ⌐ Black Pepper, ground
pinch ⌐ Cayenne Pepper, optional

○ Add above ingredients into a small bowl. Mix together. Store in an airtight container with spices for no longer than 3 months.

BROWN GROUND BEEF, PORK, CHICKEN OR TURKEY
4 SERVINGS

1 lb ➤ Meat, ground

○ Heat skillet over medium-high heat.

○ Add meat and let cook for 3-4 minutes. The meat will begin browning. Then break meat into large pieces with a spoon or spatula..

○ Continue breaking meat into smaller pieces, season as desired, and brown. Do not stir continuously, instead let it cook for a minute between each stir to let the moisture evaporate and allow the meat to brown completely without signs of pink. Serve warm or set aside for specific recipes.

NOTE: *If not needed, cool before sealing in an airtight container or a plastic bag. Refrigerate for up to 4 days. Freeze for up to 3 months.*

COOK BACON SLICES
6 TO 8 SERVINGS

1 pkg ➤ Bacon

○ Preheat oven to 375° F.

○ Line baking sheet with aluminum foil.

○ Place bacon slices on baking sheet.

○ Bake for 20-25 minutes or until desired crispness.

○ Remove from oven. Let cool for about 5 minutes.

○ Crumble bacon or cut into small pieces with kitchen scissors. Set aside to use for garnish.

NOTE: *If not needed, cool before sealing in an airtight container or a plastic bag. Use as needed or wanted within the next 10 days.*

COOK CHICKEN BREASTS
STOVE

○ Drizzle skillet with oil.

○ Heat on medium heat.

○ Once heated, add desired amount of chicken.

○ Cook for 5-7 minutes on each slide until pink begins to disappear and internal temperature reaches 165° F.

NOTE: *If not needed, cool before sealing in an airtight container or a plastic bag. Use as needed or wanted within the next 4 days.*

PREPARE JASMINE RICE
STOVE

1¼ C ⊢ Water

1 C ⊢ Rice, Jasmine

- ○ Let's make this easy. No rinsing required.
- ○ Place ingredients in saucepan and bring to a simmer on high heat.
- ○ Cover and turn to low heat for 12 minutes. Do not lift lid.
- ○ Stand 10 minutes to let the rice finish cooking.
- ○ Fluff with a fork. Serve warm.

  NOTE: *If not needed, cool before sealing in 1 cup portions, an airtight container or a plastic zip top bag, Refrigerate for no longer than 7 days. Freeze for up to 3 months.*

TOAST NUTS
OVEN

- ○ Preheat oven to 325° F.
- ○ Line baking sheet with aluminum foil.
- ○ Spread the nuts in single layer. Don't crowd or assemble them too close together.
- ○ Bake for 5–8 minutes or until desired crispness.
- ○ Remove from oven. Let cool for about 5 minutes. Serve warm.

  NOTE: *If not needed, cool before sealing in an airtight container or a plastic bag. Use as needed or wanted.*

NOTES

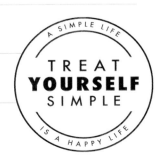

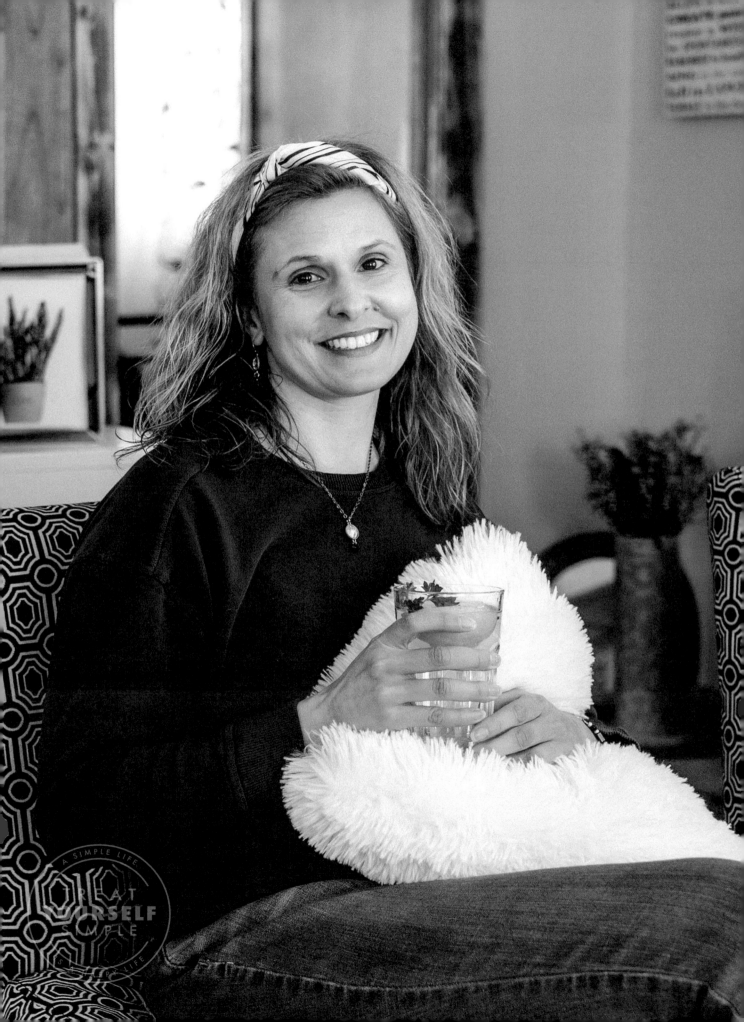

WEEK 1

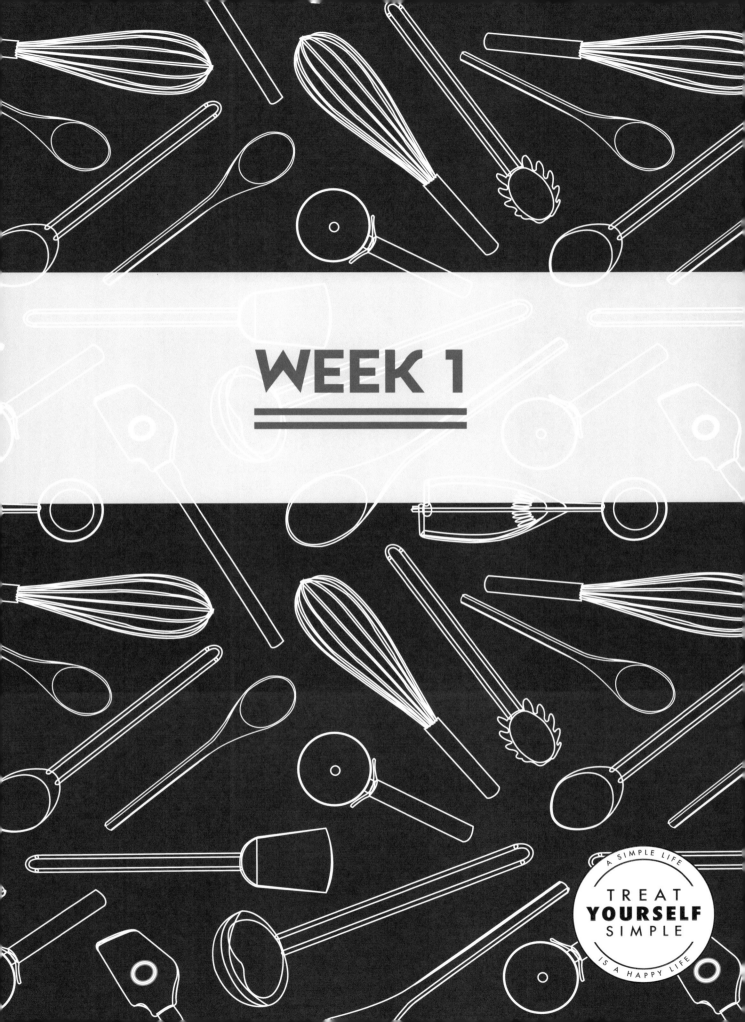

A SIMPLE LIFE
TREAT
YOURSELF
SIMPLE
IS A HAPPY LIFE

WEEK 1 MENU PLAN

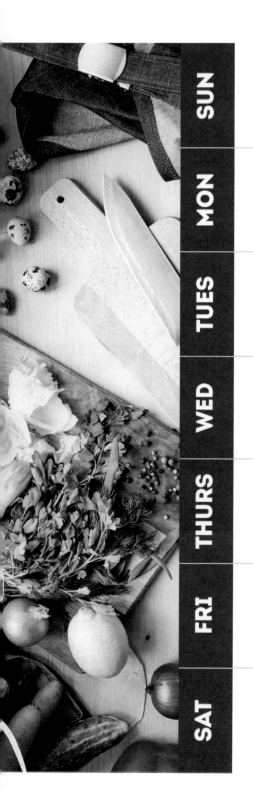

SUN

SHRIMP FAJITAS 2/1

Guacamole, Salsa and Chips
Apple Slices

MON

HONEY SOY PORK CHOPS

Jasmine Rice
Green Beans

TUES

FAJITA RICE BOWLS 2/1

Refried Beans
Apple Slices

WED

SOUTHWEST TURKEY BURGERS

Sweet Potato Disc
Coleslaw

THURS

PITA PIZZA

Fresh Salad
Pears

FRI

ROSEMARY CHICKEN

Quinoa
Brussel Sprouts

SAT

STEAK & MUSHROOMS

Mashed Cauliflower
Fresh Salad

WEEK 1 GROCERY LIST

SHRIMP FAJITAS 2/1

2	Bell Peppers, any color, fresh, sliced
optional	Cheese, Mexican, shredded
2 T	Taco Seasoning
1 T	Olive Oil
1	Onion, red, small, fresh, sliced
optional	Salsa
16 oz	Shrimp, large, raw, peeled and deveined or 4 C Salad Shrimp, half of shrimp for **Fajita Shrimp Bowls 2/1**
optional	Sour Cream
4	Tortilla Shells, 6–8", Flour or Corn

HONEY SOY PORK CHOPS

dash	Black Pepper, ground
1 T	Butter
¼ C	Broth or Stock, Chicken
¼ C	Flour, all purpose
2 t	Garlic, minced
½ T	Honey
½ T	Olive Oil
2	Pork Chops, 4 oz each
½ T	Soy Sauce

FAJITA RICE BOWLS 2/1

optional	Avocado, fresh
1 pkg	Black Beans & Rice, 6 oz package
8 oz	Shrimp Fajita mixture from **Shrimp Fajitas 2/1**
1 T	Olive Oil
optional	Sour Cream
optional	Tomatoes, cherry, fresh

SOUTHWEST TURKEY BURGERS

2	Buns, Hamburger, lightly toasted
2	Cheese, Cheddar, slices
½ t	Chili Powder
dash	Pepper, red, crushed
¼ t	Cumin, ground
2 T	Flour
optional	Ketchup, Chipotle
Dash	Kosher Salt
½ lb	Turkey, ground
¼ C	Corn, frozen

PITA PIZZA

1 T	Balsamic Vinegar
1 T	Maple Syrup
dash	Black Pepper, ground
1 C	Cheese, Mozzarella, shredded
1	Bread, Pita
1 bunch	Oregano, fresh
dash	Kosher Salt
2 t	Olive Oil
2 T	Onion, red, fresh, chopped
10	Tomatoes, cherry, fresh
½ C	Arugula, fresh

ROSEMARY CHICKEN

dash	Black Pepper, ground
2	Chicken Breasts, 4 oz each
1 T	Garlic, minced
1 T	Rosemary, fresh, chopped
dash	Kosher Salt
2 t	Lemon Juice
2 t	Mustard, yellow
1½ T	Olive Oil

STEAK & MUSHROOMS

dash	Black Pepper, ground
optional	Pepper, red, crushed
½ t	Basil, fresh, chopped
2 t	Garlic, minced
dash	Kosher Salt
½ C	Mushrooms, fresh, sliced
2 T	Olive Oil
optional	Onions, green, fresh, sliced
2	Sirloin Steaks, 4 oz each, cut into bite-sized cubes
¼ C	Soy Sauce
½ t	Thyme, dried

WEEK 1 PREP

Mince 14 Cloves Garlic ~ Honey Soy Pork Chops, Rosemary Chicken, Steak & Mushrooms

Slice 1 Red Onion ~ Shrimp Fajitas 2/1

Chop 2 T Red Onion ~ Pita Pizza

Slice 2 Bell Peppers, any color ~ Shrimp Fajitas 2/1

Shred 4 T Mexican Cheese from block ~ Shrimp Fajitas 2/1

Shred 1 C Mozzarella Cheese from block ~ Pita Pizza

WEEK 1 MAKE AHEAD

Prepare Marinade ~ Rosemary Chicken, Steak & Mushrooms

Prepare Taco Seasoning ~ Shrimp Fajitas 2/1

Cook Black Beans & Rice ~ Fajita Rice Bowls 2/1

NOTES

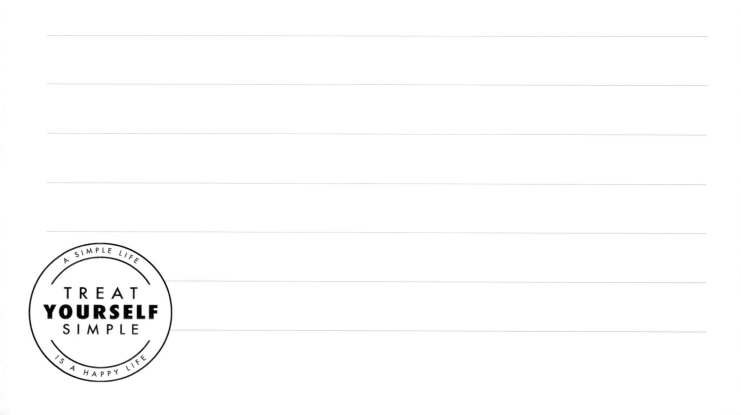

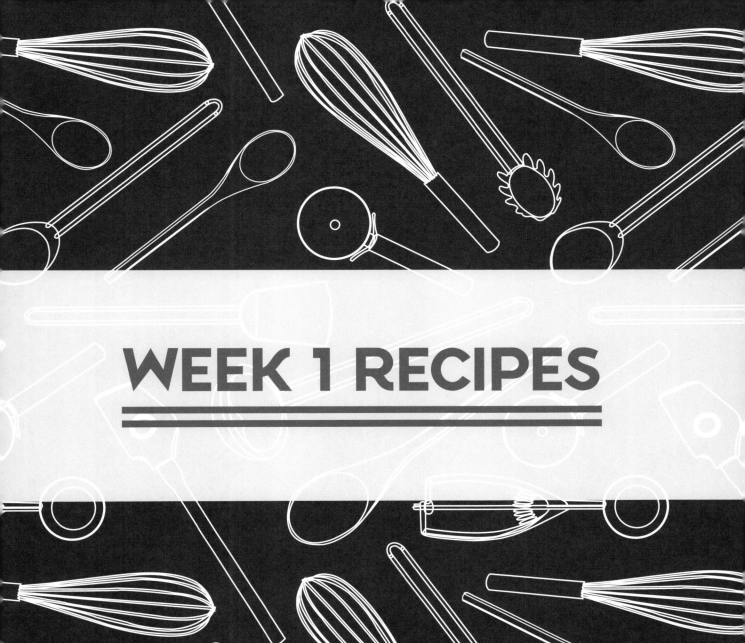

WEEK 1 RECIPES

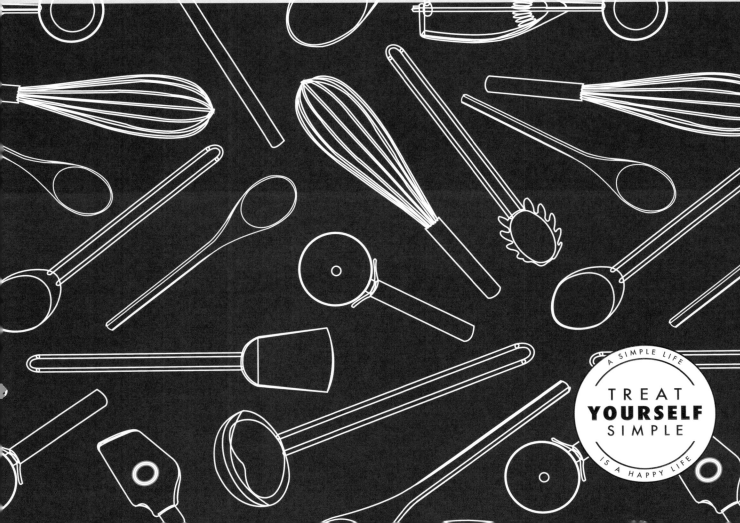

A SIMPLE LIFE
TREAT **YOURSELF** SIMPLE
IS A HAPPY LIFE

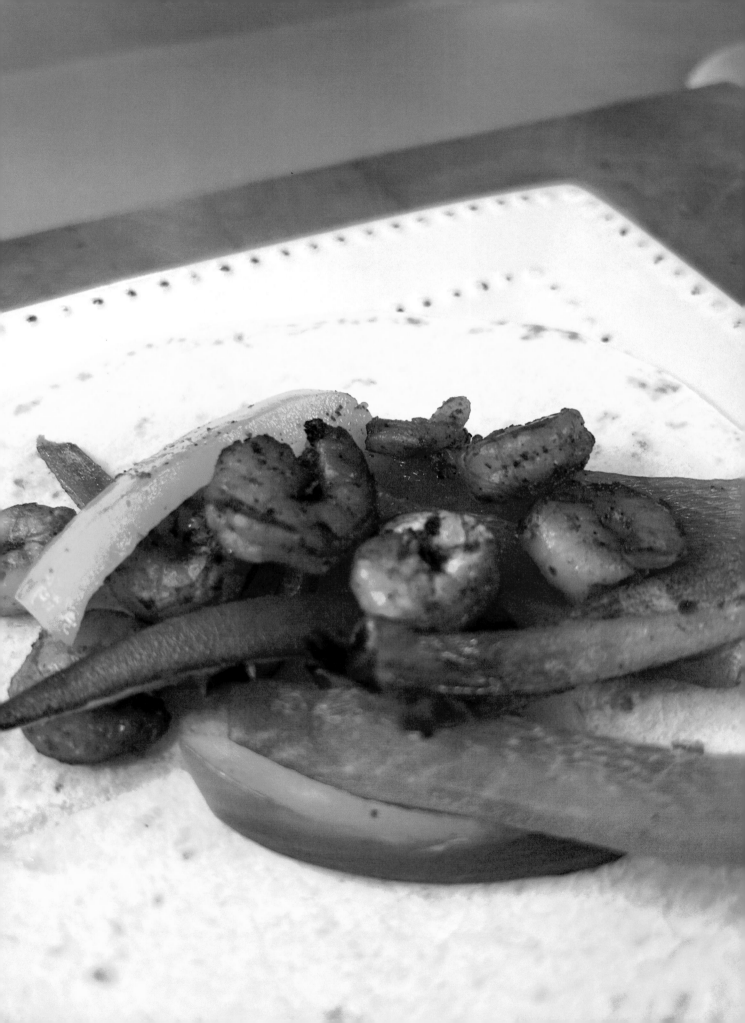

SHRIMP FAJITAS 2/1 OVEN

Please note: Makes Shrimp for Fajita Rice Bowls 2/1

Serving Size:	2 servings	Cook time:	10 minutes
Prep time:	10 minutes	Needed:	Baking sheet, medium bowl, spatula

DIRECTIONS

○ Preheat oven to 450º F. Line baking sheet with aluminum foil; coat with cooking spray; set aside.

2 T ⊳ Taco Seasoning
1 T ⊳ Olive Oil
16 oz ⊳ Shrimp, large, raw, peeled and deveined or 4 C Salad Shrimp

○ Combine taco seasoning and olive oil in medium mixing bowl. Add shrimp; toss to coat; lay out seasoned shrimp in a single layer on the prepared baking sheet.

1 ⊳ Onion, red, small, sliced
2 ⊳ Bell Peppers, any color, fresh, sliced

○ Add the above ingredients to prepared baking sheet, spreading evenly among shrimp. Bake for 8–10 minutes until internal temperature reaches 145º F.

NOTE: *Set aside half of the cooked ingredients for* **Fajita Rice Bowls 2/1** *to cool; store in a sealed container and refrigerate until ready to use.*

4 ⊳ Tortilla Shells, 6–8", Flour or Corn
optional ⊳ Sour Cream
optional ⊳ Cheese, Mexican, shredded
optional ⊳ Salsa

○ Wrap tortillas in paper towels and heat in microwave for 30 seconds; Remove, unwrap, placing 2 tortillas on two plates. Divide cooked ingredients among 4 tortillas; add optional ingredients as desired. Serve warm.

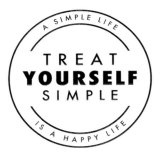

A SIMPLE LIFE
TREAT
YOURSELF
SIMPLE
IS A HAPPY LIFE

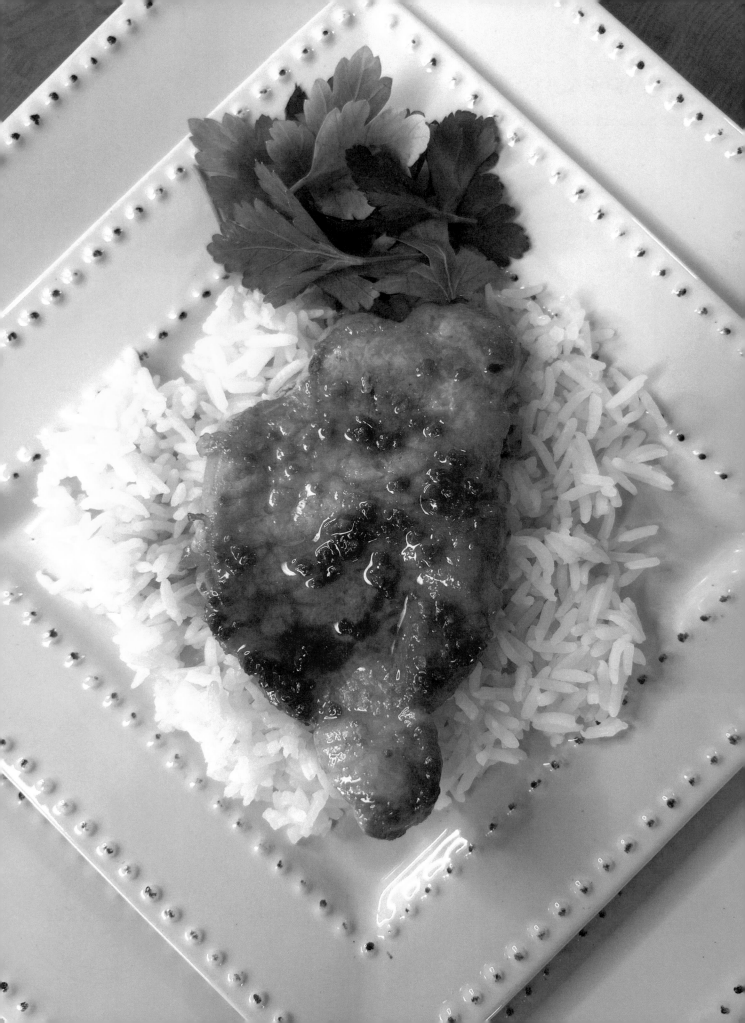

HONEY SOY PORK CHOPS   STOVE

Serving Size:	2 servings	Cook time:	15 minutes
Prep time:	5 minutes	Needed:	Shallow casserole dish, skillet, spatula

DIRECTIONS

2 ➤ Pork Chops, 4 oz each
dash ➤ Black Pepper, ground
¼ C ➤ Flour, all purpose, for dredging

○ Sprinkle the pork chops with pepper, and then dredge them in flour.

½ T ➤ Butter
½ T ➤ Olive Oil

○ Add above ingredients to skillet over medium-high heat. Once skillet is heated, add the coated pork chops. Cook for 3–4 minutes per side or until it has a nice golden crust. Take the pork chops out of the skillet and set aside.

¼ C ➤ Broth or Stock, Chicken
½ T ➤ Soy Sauce
½ T ➤ Honey
2 t ➤ Garlic, minced
½ T ➤ Butter

○ Take the skillet off the heat and add the above ingredients. Return the skillet to the heat and cook for about a minute.

○ Add the pork chops back to the skillet, reduce the heat to medium-low (or low heat if it's cast iron), cover the skillet and let the pork chops cook for 3 minutes or until it's fully cooked reaching desired doneness or 145° F.

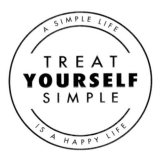

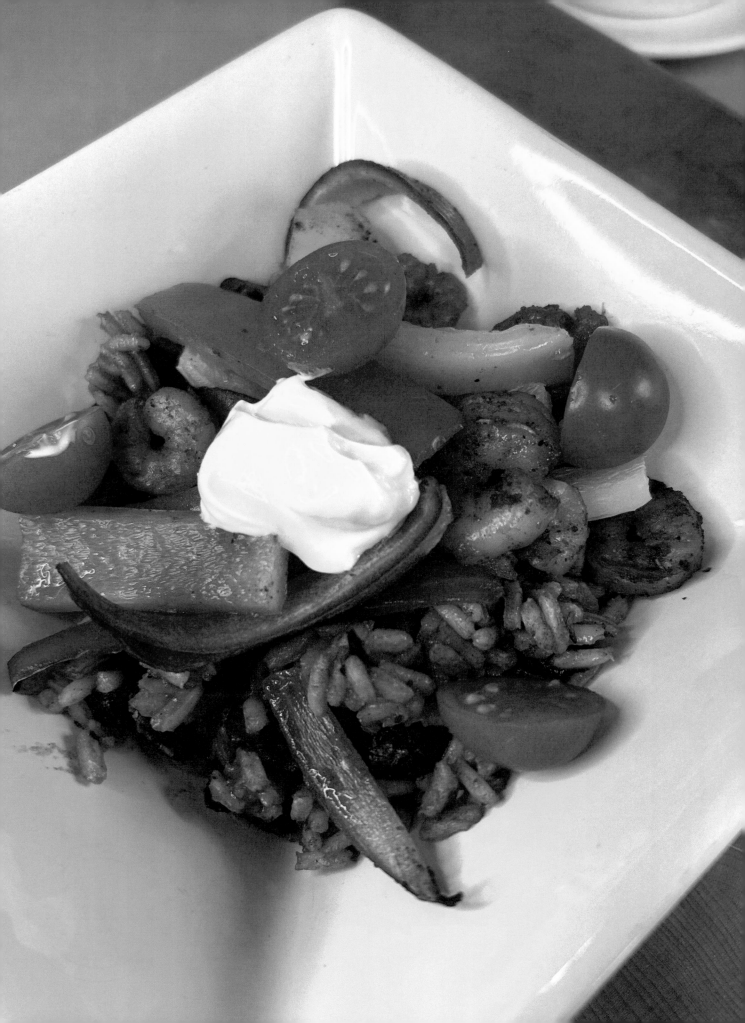

FAJITA RICE BOWLS 2/1 STOVE

Please note: Shrimp Fajita Mixture was prepared from Shrimp Fajitas 2/1

Serving Size:	2 servings	Cook time:	10 minutes
Prep time:	5 minutes	Needed:	Large skillet, medium saucepan, heat-safe spoon

DIRECTIONS

1 ➤ Black Beans & Rice, 6 oz package

○ **Can make ahead. See Make Ahead Directions.** If not already prepared, cook according to package instructions. Set aside.

½ ➤ Shrimp Fajita mixture from **Shrimp Fajitas 2/1**
1 T ➤ Olive Oil

○ Coat large skillet with olive oil over medium heat. Add black beans and rice as well as above shrimp mixture; cook for 5–8 minutes, stirring occasionally. Once heated to desired temperature. Remove from heat.

optional ➤ Avocado, fresh, sliced
optional ➤ Sour Cream
optional ➤ Tomatoes, cherry, fresh, halved

○ Divide mixture in two bowls, top with optional ingredients. Serve warm.

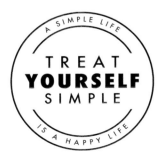

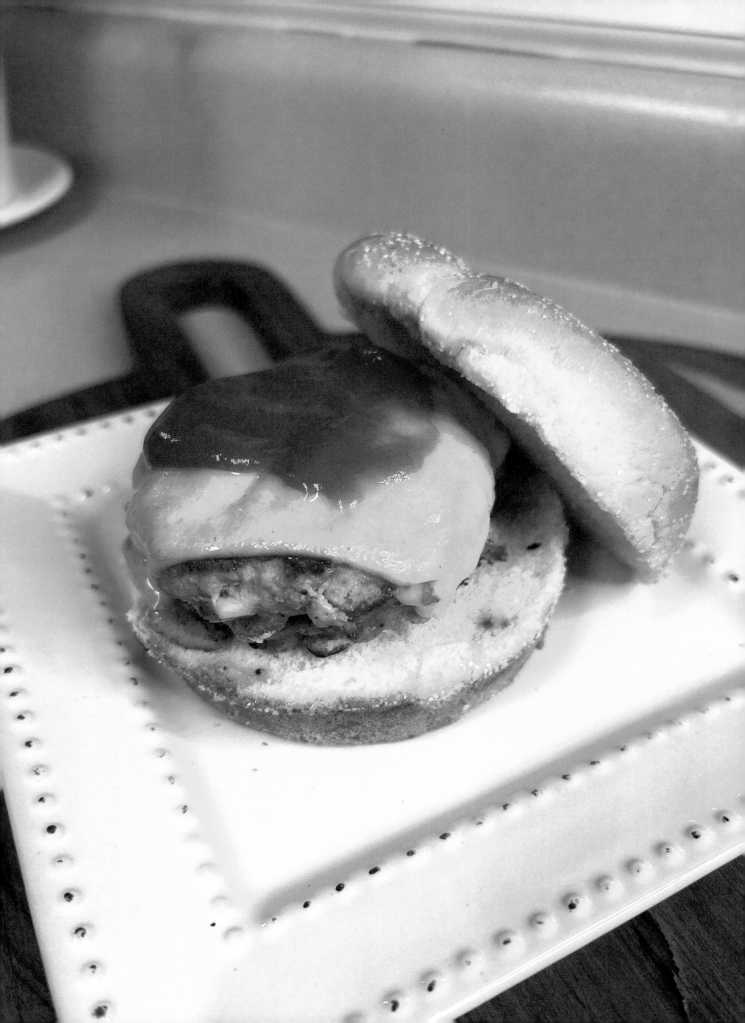

SOUTHWEST TURKEY BURGERS STOVE

Serving Size:	2 servings	Cook time:	35 minutes
Prep time:	15 minutes	Needed:	Medium bowl, large skillet, spatula

DIRECTIONS

½ t ➤ Chili Powder
dash ➤ Pepper, red, crushed
¼ t ➤ Cumin, ground
2 T ➤ Flour
dash ➤ Kosher Salt
½ lb ➤ Turkey, ground
¼ C ➤ Corn, frozen

○ Combine, in a medium mixing bowl, the above ingredients. Divide mixture into two equal portions; shaping each into a half-inch thick patty.

○ Coat a large skillet, with cooking spray on medium-high heat. Place patties; cook for 8–12 minutes, flipping at least once, until internal temperature reaches 165º F.

2 ➤ Cheese, Cheddar, slices

○ Add, to each patty, one slice of cheese to each patty; cook for 2–3 minutes until cheese melts. Remove from skillet.

2 ➤ Buns, Hamburger, lightly toasted
optional ➤ Ketchup, Chipotle

○ Wipe out skillet with a paper towel. Add, to skillet, each split roll flat part down; Lightly brown for 2–3 minutes. Remove immediately.

○ Place on two plates: Bottom of bun, patty, optional ingredients, and top of bun. Serve warm.

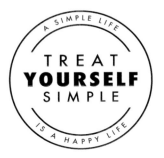

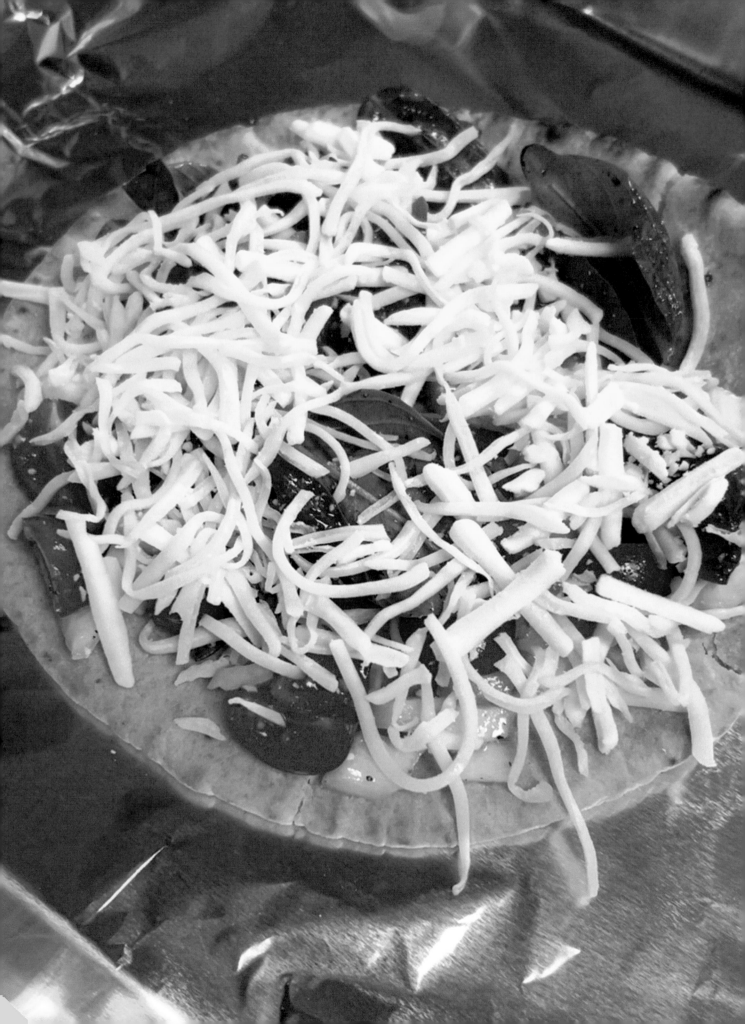

PITA PIZZA OVEN

Serving Size:	2 servings	Cook time:	15 minutes
Prep time:	15 minutes	Needed:	Medium bowl, baking sheet, measuring cup or small bowl, whisk, spatula

DIRECTIONS

○ Preheat oven to 400° F. Line baking sheet pan with aluminum foil.

1 ➤ Bread, Pita
dash ➤ Black Pepper, ground
dash ➤ Kosher Salt
2 t ➤ Olive Oil
2 T ➤ Onion, small, red, fresh chopped
1 bunch ➤ Oregano, fresh
10 ➤ Tomatoes, cherry, fresh

○ Combine above ingredients in medium bowl except pita bread.
Lay pita bread on baking sheet. Top with half of vegetable mixture.

1 C ➤ Cheese, Mozzarella, shredded

○ Sprinkle cheese over pizza mixture. Bake for 10–15 minutes
until cheese is melted.

1 T ➤ Vinegar, Balsamic
1 T ➤ Maple Syrup

○ Combine above ingredients in measuring cup or small bowl;
whisk together until blended to make balsamic glaze. Set aside.

½ C ➤ Arugula, fresh

○ Drizzle balsamic glaze on top of pizzas; top with arugula.
Cut in half, placing one each on two plates. Serve warm.

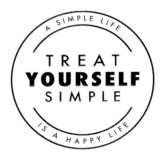

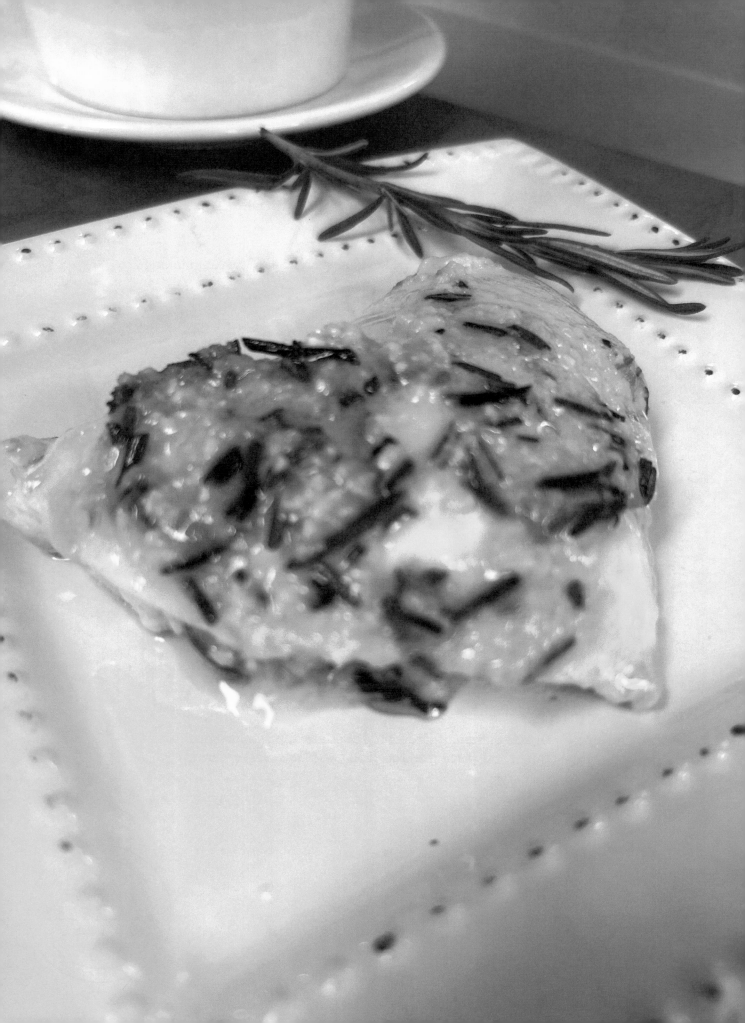

ROSEMARY CHICKEN GRILL OR OVEN

Serving Size:	2 servings	Cook time:	20–30 minutes
Prep time:	5–30 minutes	Needed:	Zip top bag or airtight container, baking sheet, spatula

dash ➤ Black Pepper, ground
2 ➤ Chicken Breasts, 4 oz
1 T ➤ Garlic, minced
1 T ➤ Rosemary, fresh, chopped
dash ➤ Kosher Salt
2 t ➤ Lemon Juice
2 t ➤ Mustard, yellow
1½ T ➤ Olive Oil

DIRECTIONS

MARINADE

○ **Can make ahead. See Make Ahead Directions.** If not already prepared, Combine, in a zip top bag, the above ingredients. Add chicken. Seal bag and rub marinade over the chicken or place in airtight container, rubbing marinade on chicken. Seal container. Place into refrigerator for 30 minutes up to one day.

GRILL

○ Preheat grill to medium-high heat. Remove chicken from marinade; discard marinade. Place chicken on grill; cook for 8–12 minutes, flipping at least once, until the internal temperature reaches 165º F. Remove from heat and let rest for 5 minutes before slicing and serving. Serve warm.

OVEN

○ Preheat oven 350º F. Spray baking sheet with cooking spray. Remove chicken from marinade; discard marinade. Place chicken on baking sheet. Bake for 20–25 minutes until the internal temperature reaches 165º F.

○ Remove from oven and let rest for 5 minutes before slicing and serving. Serve warm.

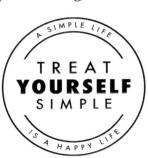
A SIMPLE LIFE
TREAT
YOURSELF
SIMPLE
IS A HAPPY LIFE

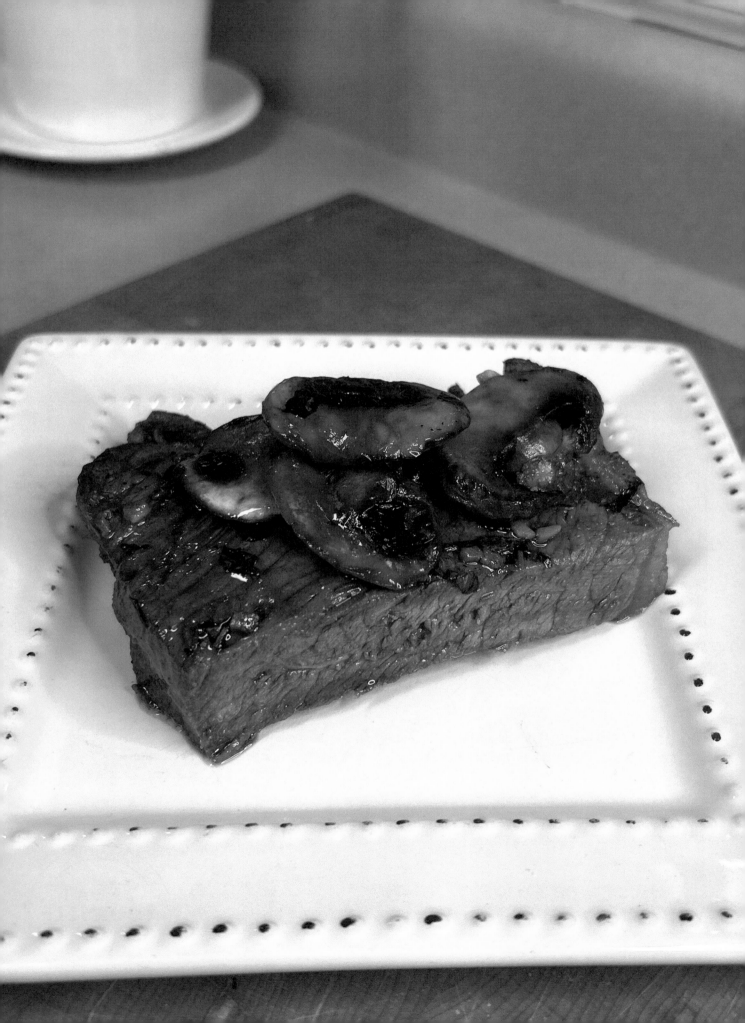

STEAK & MUSHROOMS GRILL OR OVEN

Serving Size:	2 servings	Cook time:	20 minutes
Prep time:	30 minutes	Needed:	Zip top bag, foil packets, baking sheet, spatula

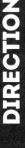

DIRECTIONS

dash ➤ Black Pepper, ground
½ t ➤ Basil, fresh, chopped
2 t ➤ Garlic, minced
dash ➤ Kosher Salt
½ C ➤ Mushrooms, fresh, sliced
2 T ➤ Olive Oil
2 ➤ Sirloin Steaks, 4 oz each, cut into bite-sized cubes
¼ C ➤ Soy Sauce
½ t ➤ Thyme, dried

MARINADE

○ **Can make ahead. See Make Ahead Directions.** If not already prepared, combine above ingredients in a zip top bag. Add steak. Seal bag and rub marinade over the steak. Place in refrigerator for 15–30 minutes.

optional ➤ Pepper, red, crushed
optional ➤ Onions, green, fresh, sliced

GRILL

○ Preheat grill on medium heat. Remove steak from marinade; discard marinade. Divide, in foil packets, steak and mushrooms; close packet. Place on grill; cook for 20 minutes, flipping packet over once, until internal temperature reaches 145° F. Remove from heat. Divide steak mixture and optional ingredients. Serve warm.

OVEN

○ Preheat oven to 400° F. Remove steak from marinade; discard marinade. Divide, in foil packets, steak and mushrooms; close packet. Bake for 10–12 minutes or until desired doneness is reached. Let mixture rest for 5 minutes before slicing. Divide steak mixture and optional ingredients. Serve warm.

A SIMPLE LIFE
TREAT
YOURSELF
SIMPLE
IS A HAPPY LIFE

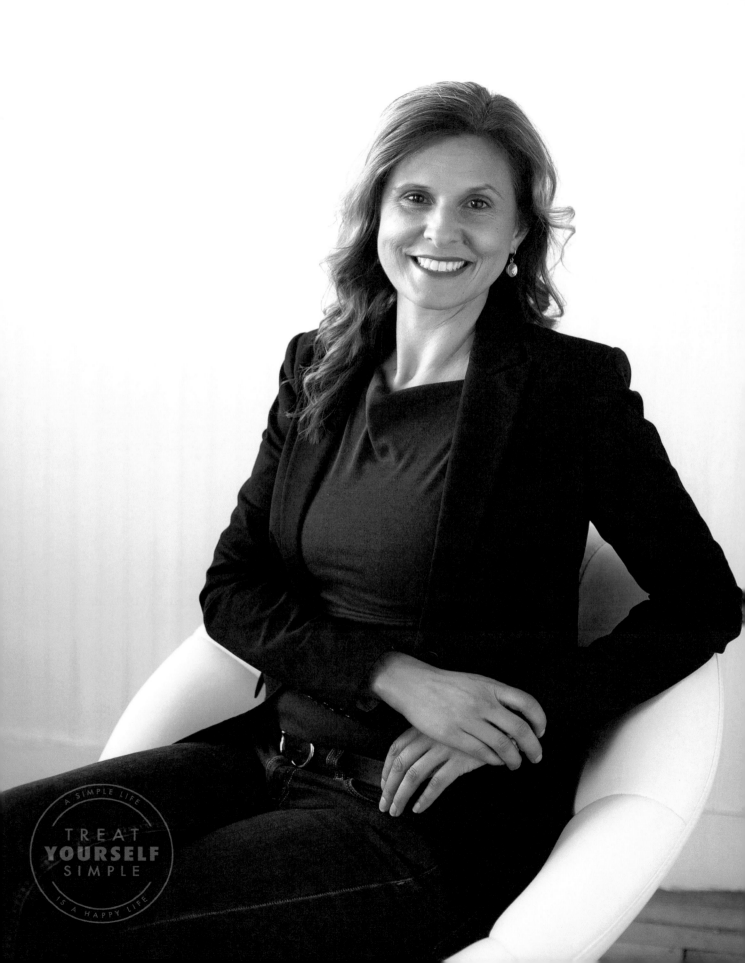

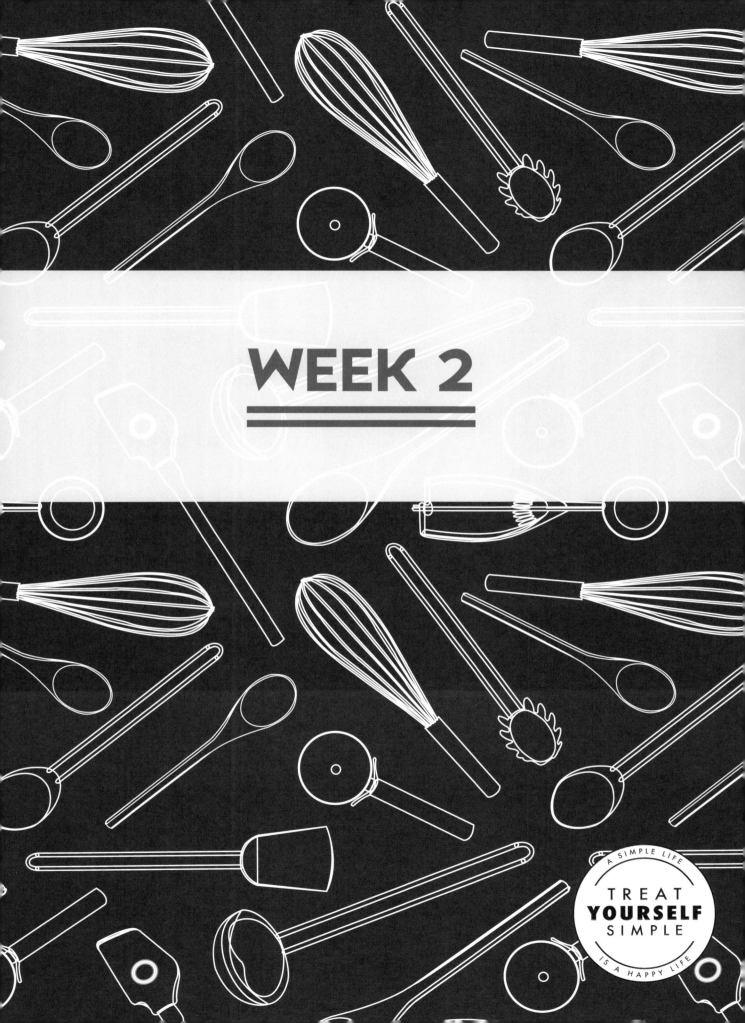

WEEK 2

WEEK 2 MENU PLAN

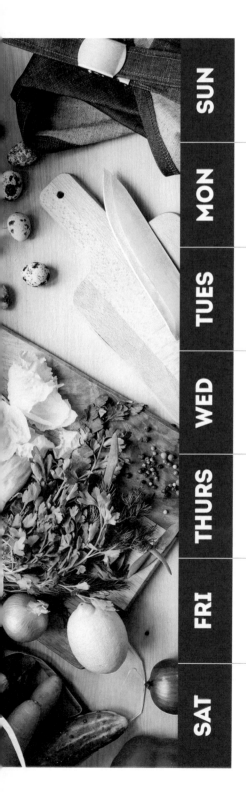

SUN

SLOW COOKER CHICKEN 2/1
Quinoa
Brussel Sprouts

MON

PERFECT POTATO SOUP
Sweet Potato Disc
Cinnamon Apples

TUES

PARMESAN CHICKEN SANDWICH
Fresh Salad
Pears

WED

CHICKEN QUESADILLAS 2/1
Guacamole & Tortilla Chips
Orange Slices

THURS

STUFFED PEPPERS
Cottage Cheese
Pears

FRI

SALMON CHOWDER
Coleslaw
Cinnamon Apples

SAT

CIDER BRAISED CHICKEN
Fresh Salad
Pears

WEEK 2 GROCERY LIST

BY MEAL

SLOW COOKER CHICKEN 2/1

1	Chicken, whole, half for **Chicken Quesadillas**
3 T	Garlic, minced
2	Rosemary, fresh, bunches
1 T	Kosher Salt
2	Lemons, fresh, sliced

PERFECT POTATO SOUP

1 slice	Bacon, crumbled, or 1 T Real Bacon Bits/Crumbles
dash	Black Pepper, ground
½ C	Carrots, chopped
1 stalk	Celery, fresh, chopped
¼ C	Cheese, Colby Jack, shredded
¾ t	Flour
dash	Cream, heavy
½ t	Parsley, fresh, chopped
dash	Kosher Salt
¾ t	Flour
¼ C	Milk
1 T	Olive Oil
¼ C	Onion, sweet, chopped
2	Potatoes, Russet, small, diced
2 C	Broth, Vegetable

PARMESAN CHICKEN SANDWICHES

⅛ t	Black Pepper, ground
¾ C	Breadcrumbs
2	Chicken Breasts, 4 oz each
1	Egg, large
½ C	Flour, all-purpose
2	Buns, Kaiser
⅛ t	Kosher Salt
1 T	Olive Oil
⅓ C	Marinara or other meatless Pasta Sauce, warmed
3 T	Cheese, Parmesan/Romano, grated
2	Cheese, Provolone, slices

CHICKEN QUESADILLAS 2/1

1 pkg	Black Beans & Rice, 6 oz
2 C	Chicken, shredded, from **Slow Cooker Chicken 2/1**
1 t	Cilantro, fresh, chopped
½ C	Corn, frozen
¼ C	Cheese, Mexican, shredded
1 T	Olive Oil
2 T	Onion, sweet, chopped
8	Tortillas, 6" or 8", Flour or Corn

STUFFED PEPPERS

½ lb	Beef, ground
2	Bell Peppers, any color, fresh
¼ t	Black Pepper, ground
½ C	Cheese, Colby Jack, shredded
½ can	Tomatoes, diced, 14 oz can
¼ t	Basil, fresh, chopped
¼ t	Garlic, minced
½ t	Oregano, fresh, chopped
¼ t	Kosher Salt
1 C	Onion, sweet, chopped
½ C	Rice, Jasmine
½ t	Worcestershire Sauce

SALMON CHOWDER

1 T	Olive Oil or Butter, melted
1	Onion, diced, or 2 Leeks, sliced or 2 fat Shallots, diced
1	Fennel bulb, small, diced
¾ C	Celery, chopped
1 T	Garlic, minced
1 t	Celery Seed
½ t	Thyme, dried or 2 t fresh
½ t	Paprika
3 C	Stock, Chicken
¾ lb	Potatoes, baby, thinly sliced, ¼" thick
1 t	Kosher Salt
1	Bay leaf
¾ C	Milk
8 oz	Salmon, skinless. (or OK to sub other fish like Cod or Shrimp), cut into bite-sized pieces
optional	Lemon wedges
optional	Dill or Tarragon, fresh

CIDER BRAISED CHICKEN

BY MEAL

1	Apple, medium, cut into wedges
2 slices	Bacon, cut into pieces
1 C	Brussels Sprouts, fresh, trimmed, halved
2	Chicken Breasts, 4 oz each
6 oz	Hard Cider
1 T	Thyme, fresh, chopped
½ t	Kosher Salt
1 T	Mustard, yellow

WEEK 2 PREP

Mince 14 Garlic Cloves ~ Slow Cooker Chicken 2/1, Stuffed Peppers, Salmon Chowder

Chop 2 ½ Sweet Onions ~ Perfect Potato Soup, Stuffed Peppers, Salmon Chowder, Chicken Quesadillas 2/1

Chop 4 stalks Celery ~ Perfect Potato Soup, Salmon Chowder

Dice 1 small Fennel Bulb ~ Salmon Chowder

Cut 8 oz Salmon into bite-sized pieces ~ Salmon Chowder

Chop 1 medium Carrot ~ Perfect Potato Soup

Shred ¼ C Colby Jack Cheese from block ~ Perfect Potato Soup

Shred 2 C Chicken from Slow Cooker Chicken 2/1 ~ Chicken Quesadillas 2/1

WEEK 2 MAKE AHEAD

Prepare 3 slices Bacon ~ Perfect Potato Soup, Cider Braised Chicken

Cook 1 C Jasmine Rice ~ Stuffed Peppers

NOTES

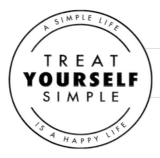

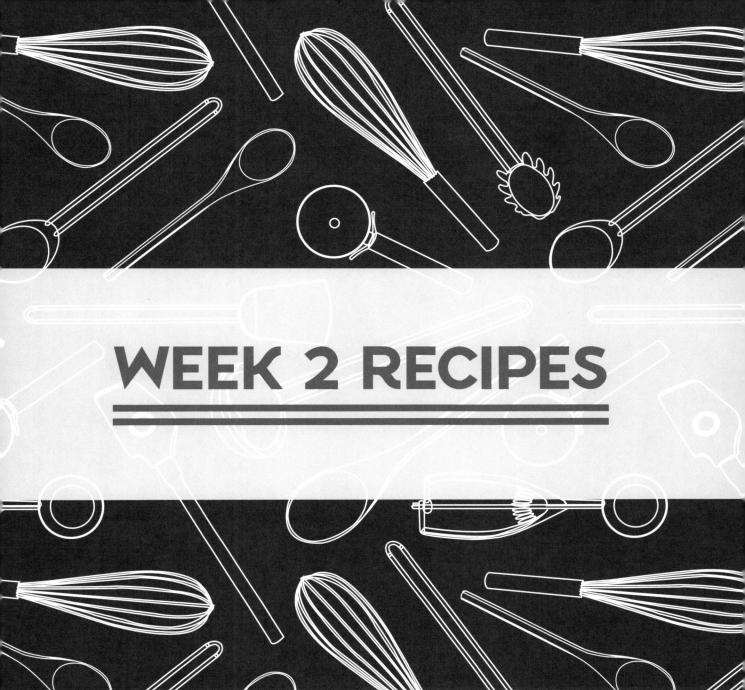

WEEK 2 RECIPES

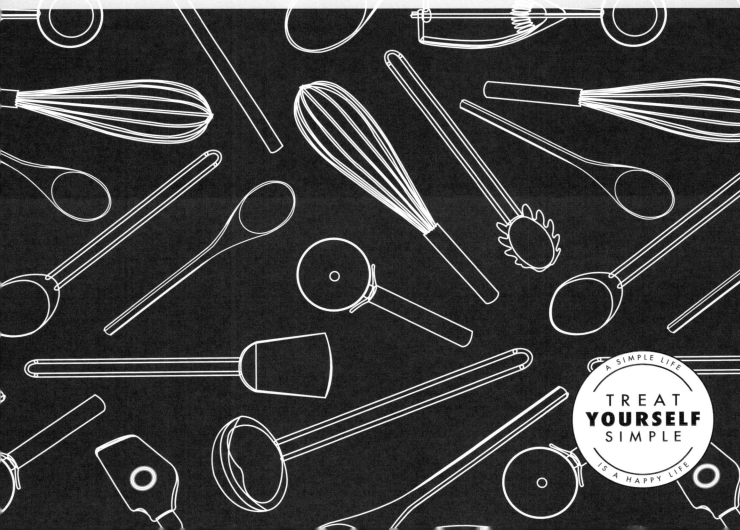

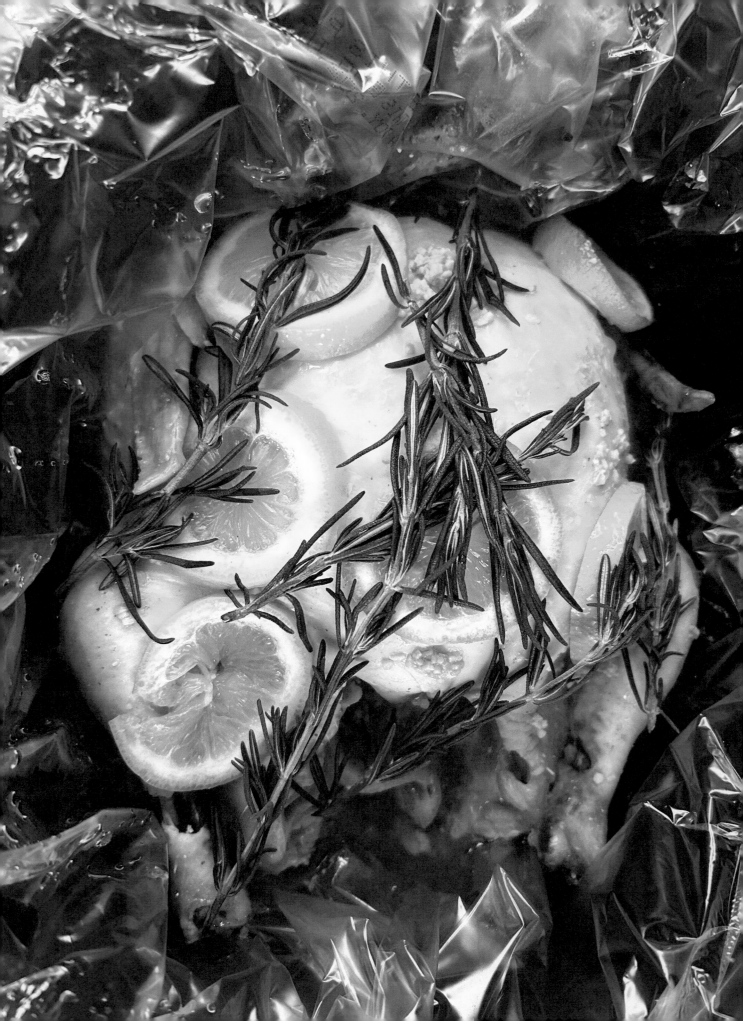

SLOW COOKER CHICKEN 2/1 SLOW COOKER

Please note: Makes Chicken for Chicken Quesadillas 2/1

Serving Size:	2 servings	Cook time:	4 hours 15 minutes
Prep time:	10 minutes	Needed:	Slow cooker, slow cooker liner, plate, tongs

DIRECTIONS

1 ➤ Chicken, whole
3 T ➤ Garlic, minced
1 T ➤ Kosher Salt
2 ➤ Lemons, fresh, sliced

○ Line slow cooker with a slow cooker liner. Layer 1 t garlic and one-third of the lemon slices in the slower cooker bottom. Rinse and pat dry the whole chicken; stuff inside of chicken with 1 t garlic and one-third of the lemon slices. Season chicken with salt, inside and out.

2 ➤ Rosemary, fresh, bunches

○ Lay chicken in the slow cooker. Top with remaining 1 t garlic, one-third of the lemon slices, and fresh rosemary. Cook on high for 4 hours until internal temperature reaches 165º F.

○ Turn slower cooker off; let chicken rest for about 15 minutes. Remove chicken from slow cooker and carve. Serve warm.

○ Shred and set aside 2 cups of chicken for **Chicken Quesadillas 2/1.** Cool. Store in an airtight container. Refrigerate for 7–10 days.

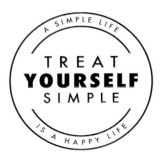

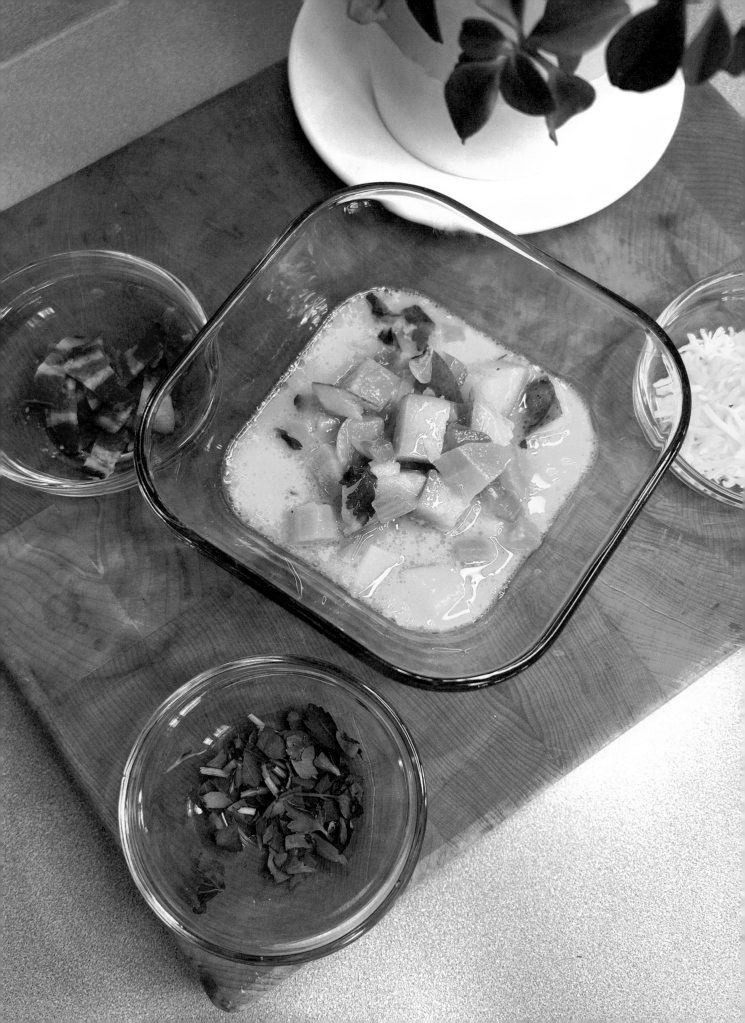

PERFECT POTATO SOUP STOVE

Serving Size:	2 servings	Cook time:	15–20 minutes
Prep time:	10 minutes	Needed:	Baking sheet, plate, paper towels, medium saucepan, small bowl, tongs, heat-safe spoon

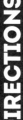

DIRECTIONS

1 T ⌁ Olive Oil
¼ C ⌁ Onion, sweet, chopped
½ C ⌁ Carrots, chopped
¼ C ⌁ Celery, chopped
2 ⌁ Potatoes, Russet, small, diced
dash ⌁ Kosher Salt
dash ⌁ Black Pepper, ground

○ Coat medium saucepan with olive oil over medium heat. Add above ingredients, stir and cook for 2 minutes. Add above ingredients and season. Cook for 5 minutes, stirring frequently.

2 C ⌁ Broth, Vegetable

○ Add broth to same pan. Bring it to a gentle boil. Reduce to medium heat; cook for 5 minutes, stirring occasionally so the vegetables don't stick to the bottom.

¼ C ⌁ Milk
¾ t ⌁ Flour

○ In the meantime, whisk together above ingredients in small bowl. Add to the soup, stirring to combine. Cook for an additional 5 minutes or until the potatoes are tender.

dash ⌁ Cream, heavy

○ Stir in cream to already heated soup.

1 slice ⌁ Bacon or 1 T Real Bacon Bits/Crumbles

○ **Can make ahead. See Make Ahead Directions.** Preheat oven to 375º F. Line baking sheet with aluminum foil. Place bacon slices on baking sheet. Bake for 25 minutes. Remove from oven and baking sheet. Line paper towels on a plate. Place cooked bacon slices on paper towels to drain grease. Let cool for about 5 minutes. Crumble bacon or cut into small pieces with kitchen scissors. Set aside for garnish. Refrigerate extra for 7–10 days to use for other meals.

¼ C ⌁ Cheese, Colby Jack, shredded
½ t ⌁ Parsley, fresh, chopped

○ Garnish with above ingredients. Serve warm.

A SIMPLE LIFE
TREAT
YOURSELF
SIMPLE
IS A HAPPY LIFE

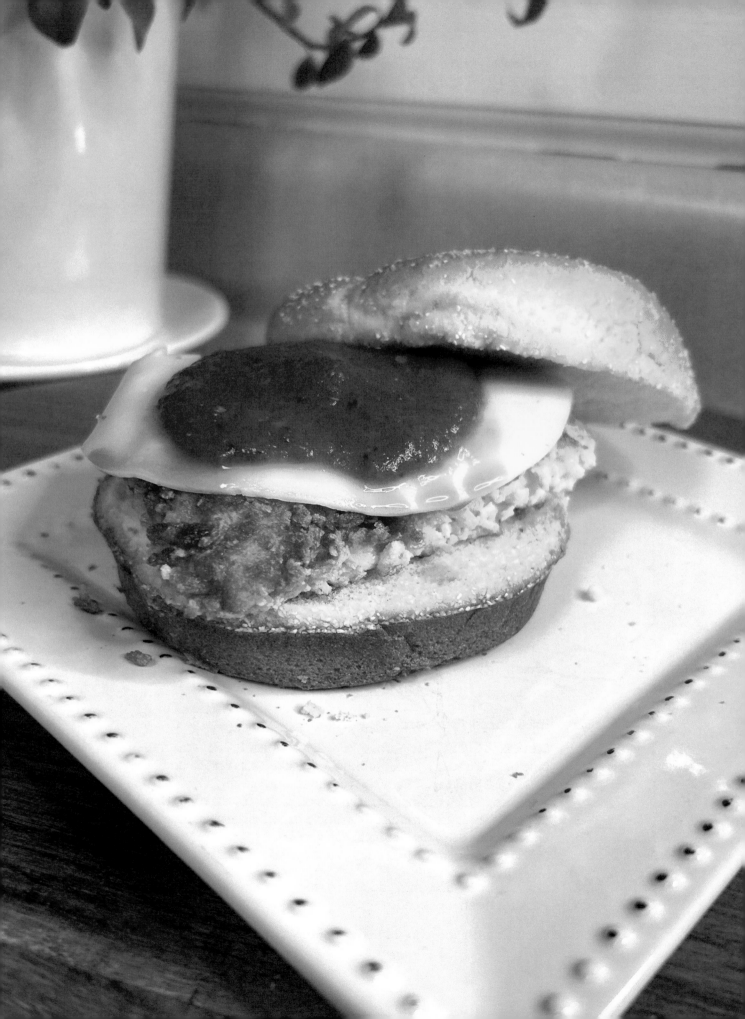

PARMESAN CHICKEN SANDWICHES STOVE

Serving Size:	2 servings	Cook time:	15 minutes
Prep time:	5 minutes	Needed:	Plate, two medium bowls, skillet, spatula

DIRECTIONS

½ C ➤ Flour, all-purpose
⅛ t ➤ Kosher Salt
⅛ t ➤ Black Pepper, ground

○ Place above ingredients in bowl, set aside.

1 ➤ Egg, large

○ Add egg in separate mixing bowl. Whisk egg yolk and egg white together. Set aside.

¾ C ➤ Breadcrumbs, any type
3 T ➤ Cheese, Parmesan/Romano, grated
2 ➤ Chicken Breasts, 4 oz each

○ Toss above ingredients together in medium bowl. Set aside.

○ Dredge chicken in flour to coat both sides; shake off excess. Coat with egg. Then dredge in crumb mixture. Coat both slides as best as you can. Discard remaining ingredients in dishes.

1 T ➤ Olive Oil

○ In large skillet, heat oil over medium heat. Add coated chicken; cook 4-5 minutes per side until golden brown and chicken is no longer pink or internal temperature reaches 165° F.

2 ➤ Cheese, Provolone, slices
⅓ C ➤ Marina or other meatless Pasta Sauce, warmed

○ Top chicken with above ingredients. Serve on buns topped with one cheese slice and sauce.

2 ➤ Buns, Kaiser, warmed

○ Add chicken to buns. Serve warm.

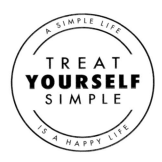

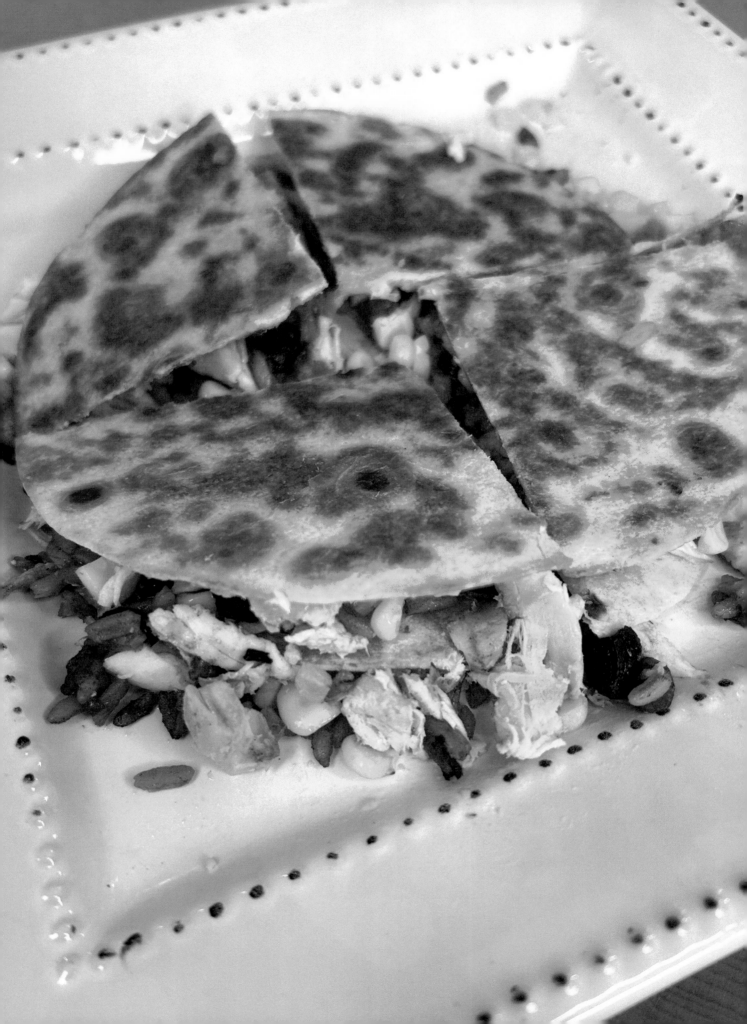

CHICKEN QUESADILLAS 2/1 STOVE

Please note: Chicken was prepared from Slow Cooker Chicken 2/1

Serving Size:	2 servings	Cook time:	20 minutes
Prep time:	5 minutes	Needed:	Two large skillets, medium mixing bowl, olive oil, spoon, spatula

DIRECTIONS

1 ➢ Black Beans & Rice, 6 oz package

○ **Can make ahead. See Make Ahead Directions.** If not already prepared, prepare black beans and rice according to package instructions. Set aside.

1 T ➢ Olive Oil
2 T ➢ Onion, sweet, chopped
2 C ➢ Chicken, shredded, from **Slow Cooker Chicken 2/1**
½ C ➢ Corn, frozen

○ Coat skillet with olive oil over medium heat. Sauté onion until translucent, about 3–5 minutes. Add the above ingredients to skillet; stir in, cooking for 5–8 minutes or until desired temperature is reached. Remove from heat, add mixture into medium mixing bowl. Set aside.

¼ C ➢ Cheese, Mexican, shredded
1 t ➢ Cilantro, fresh, chopped
8 ➢ Tortilla Shells, 6–8", Flour or Corn

○ Coat same skillet used above with olive oil, over medium heat. Layer one tortilla shell in skillet; spread evenly, one-quarter of the chicken mixture, one-quarter of the cheese, one-quarter of the cilantro and top with one shell. Lightly brush, top tortilla shell, with olive oil.

○ Heat second skillet on medium heat; place on top of tortilla for 3–4 minutes until cheese melts. Remove top skillet and quesadilla. Repeat above process until mixture is used up. Cut quesadillas into quarters. Serve warm.

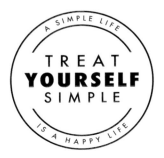
A SIMPLE LIFE
TREAT
YOURSELF
SIMPLE
IS A HAPPY LIFE

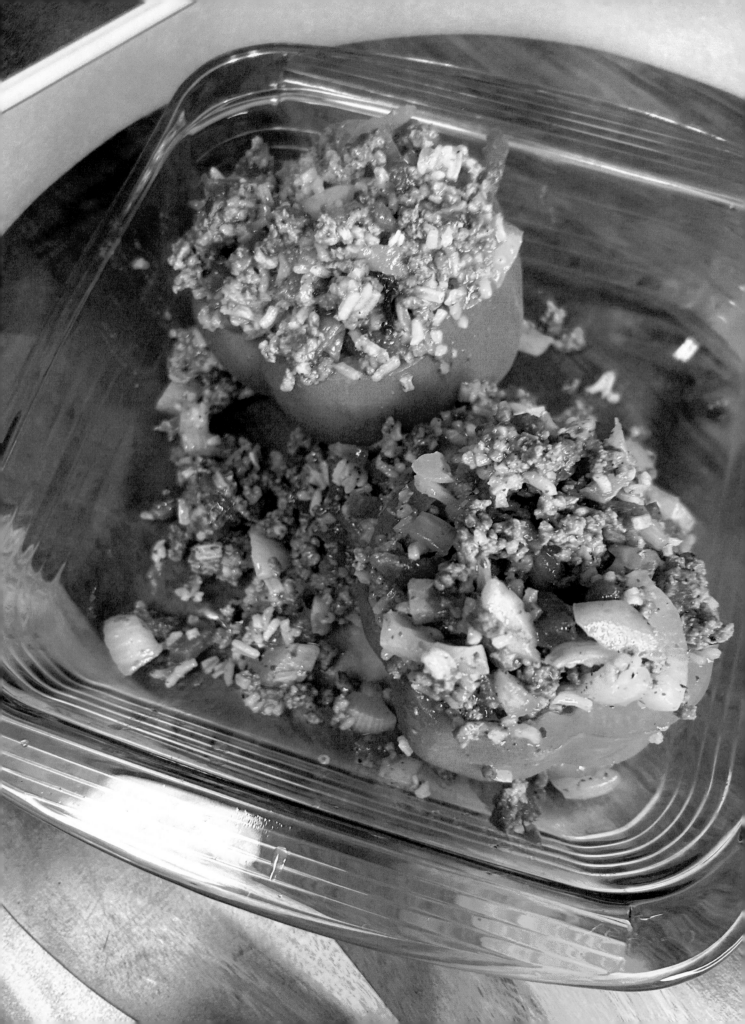

STUFFED PEPPERS OVEN

Serving Size:	2 servings	Cook time:	35 minutes
Prep time:	15 minutes	Needed:	Large pot, large skillet, spatula or heat-safe spoon, casserole dish

DIRECTIONS

○ Preheat oven to 400° F

½ C ➤ Rice, Jasmine

○ **Can make ahead. See Make Ahead Directions.** If not already prepared, cook rice according to package instructions. Set aside.

2 ➤ Bell Peppers, any color, fresh, tops removed and seeded

○ Place in a casserole dish cut side up. Set aside.

½ lb ➤ Beef, ground
1 C ➤ Onion, sweet, chopped
½ t ➤ Oregano, fresh, chopped
½ t ➤ Worcestershire Sauce
¼ t ➤ Black Pepper, ground
¼ t ➤ Kosher Salt
¼ t ➤ Garlic, minced
¼ t ➤ Basil, fresh, chopped
½ can ➤ Tomatoes, diced, drained; save the juice, 14 oz can

○ Coat a large skillet with olive oil over medium heat. Sauté garlic and onion for 3–5 minutes until translucent; add the rest of the above ingredients, mixing well; brown for 8–10 minutes, breaking the meat apart, until the reaches an internal temperature of 160º F. Add cooked rice; mix well. Remove from heat.

➤ Saved tomato juice
½ C ➤ Cheese, Colby Jack, shredded

○ Fill peppers with beef mixture; pour saved tomato juice over the filled/prepared peppers. Bake for 20 minutes. Remove from oven; add shredded cheese to the top of each pepper; return to oven for 5 minutes until cheese melts. Serve warm.

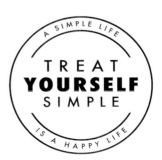

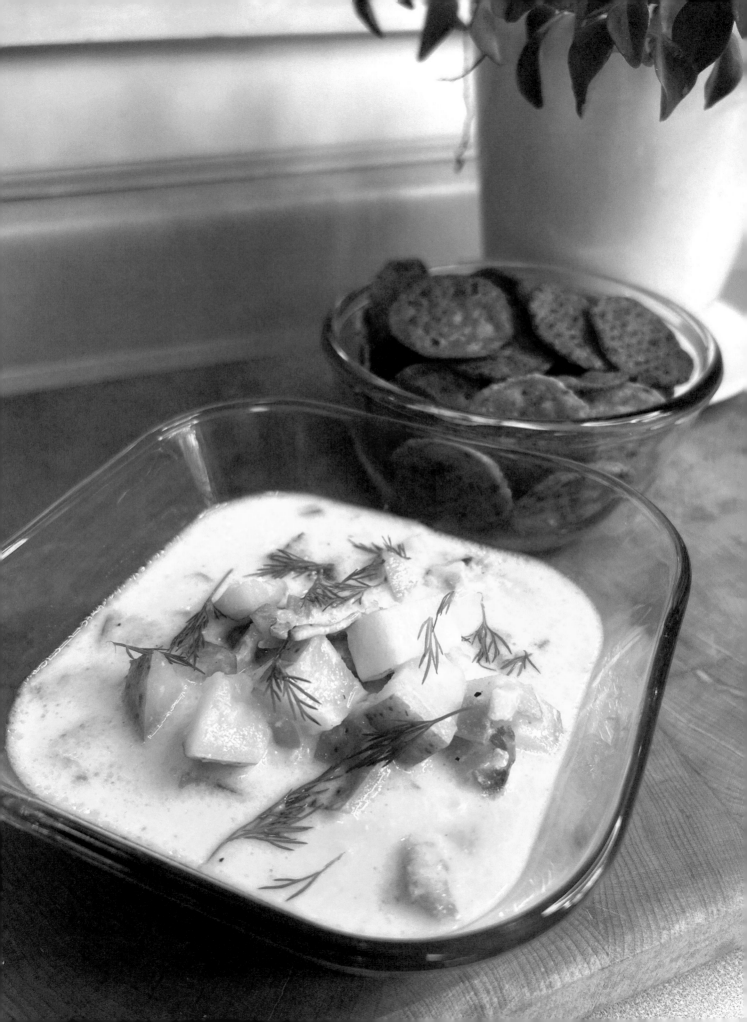

SALMON CHOWDER STOVE

Serving Size:	4 servings	Cook time:	20 minutes
Prep time:	10 minutes	Needed:	Large pot, heat-safe spoon

DIRECTIONS

1 T ➤ Olive Oil or Butter, melted
1 ➤ Onion, diced or 2 Leeks, sliced or 2 fat Shallots
1 ➤ Fennel bulb, small, diced
¾ C ➤ Celery, chopped

○ Add above ingredients and saute 5–6 minutes.

1 T ➤ Garlic, minced
1 t ➤ Celery Seed
½ t ➤ Thyme, dried, or 2 t fresh
½ t ➤ Paprika

○ Add above ingredients and saute 2 more minutes.

3 C ➤ Stock, Chicken
¾ lb ➤ Potatoes, baby, thinly sliced, ¼" thick
1 t ➤ Kosher Salt
1 ➤ Bay leaf
¾ C ➤ Milk

○ Add above ingredients, stir. Bring to a simmer, cover and simmer
over medium-low heat until tender, about 8–10 minutes
(check at 7 mins, be careful to not overcook).

8 oz ➤ Salmon, skinless. (or OK to sub other fish like Cod or Shrimp),
cut into bite-sized pieces

○ Add the above ingredient, gently poaching it in the soup for just about
2–5 minutes. Turn heat off.

optional ➤ Lemon wedges
optional ➤ Dill or Tarragon, fresh

○ Divide between two bowls.
Garnish with above ingredients. Serve warm.

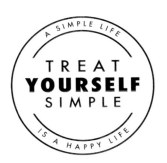

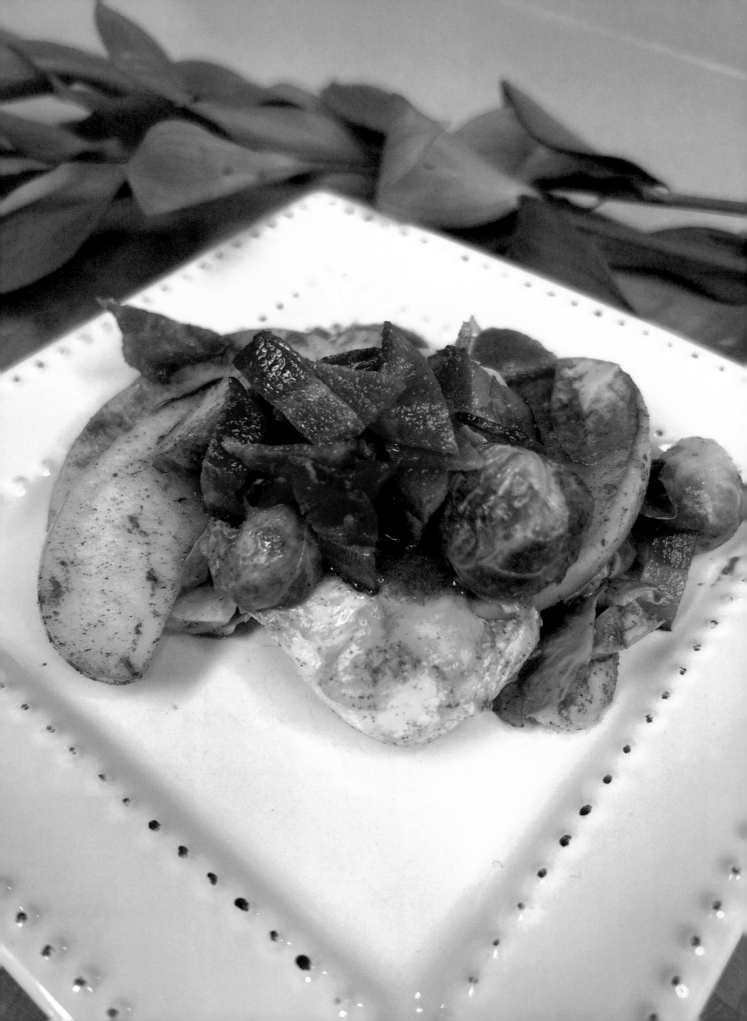

CIDER BRAISED CHICKEN OVEN/STOVE

Serving Size:	2 servings	Cook time:	25 minutes
Prep time:	10 minutes	Needed:	Baking sheet, large skillet, tongs

DIRECTIONS

2 slices ➤ Bacon, cut into pieces

○ **Can make ahead. See Make Ahead Directions.** Preheat oven to 375° F.
Line baking sheet with aluminum foil. Place bacon slices on baking sheet.
Bake for 25 minutes. Remove from oven and baking sheet.
Line paper towels to a plate. Place cooked bacon slices on paper towels
to drain grease. Let cool for about 5 minutes.

○ Crumble bacon or cut into small pieces with kitchen scissors.
Set aside to use for garnish. Refrigerate any extra for 7–10 days
and use for other meals.

1 T ➤ Olive Oil
2 ➤ Chicken Breasts, 4 oz each
1 ➤ Apple, medium, cut into wedges

○ Coat skillet with olive oil over medium heat. Coat skillet with oil.
Add chicken; cook for 4 minutes per side. Add apples to the skillet,
cooking an additional 4 minutes or until apples are browned on both sides
remove from skillet; set aside chicken and apple mixture.

6 oz ➤ Hard Cider
1 T ➤ Thyme, fresh, chopped
1 T ➤ Mustard, yellow
½ t ➤ Kosher Salt

○ In same skillet. add the above ingredients on medium heat bringing sauce to
boiling; reduce heat. Return chicken to skillet; cover and simmer 5 minutes.

1 C ➤ Brussels Sprouts, fresh, trimmed, halved

○ Add above ingredient to same skillet; cover and cook 5 minutes.
Add cooked chicken and apples; cook, uncovered, 3–5 minutes .

Divide chicken, brussels sprouts, and apples among
shallow bowls. Spoon cider mixture over top.
Sprinkle each serving with bacon. Serve warm.

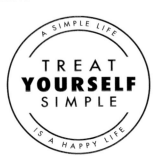

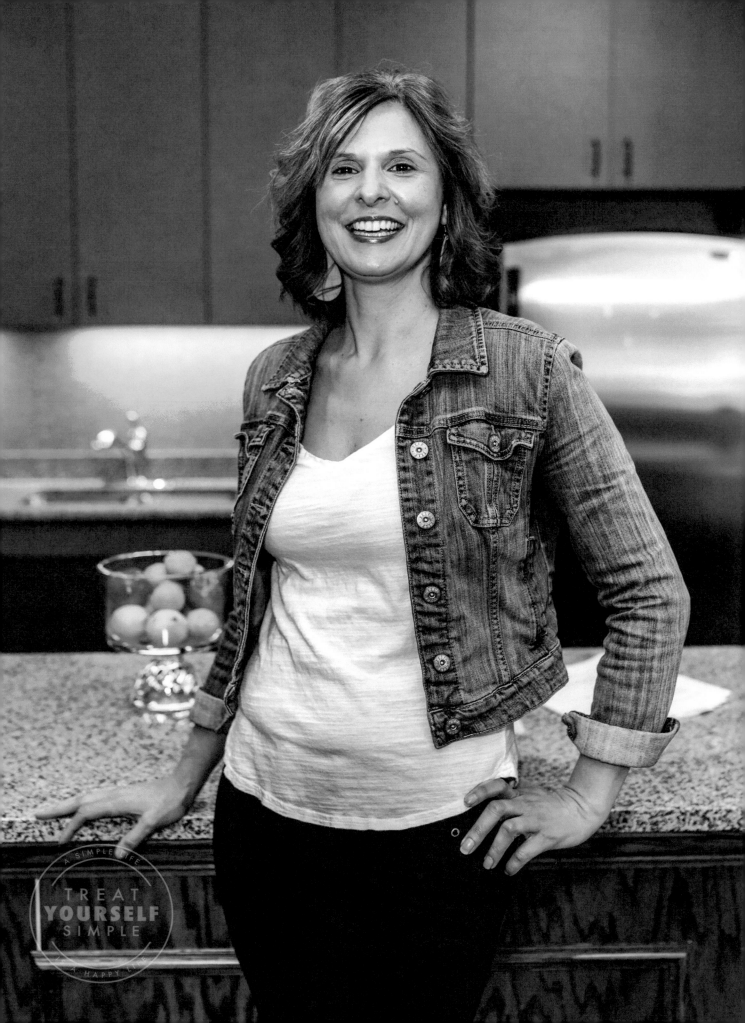

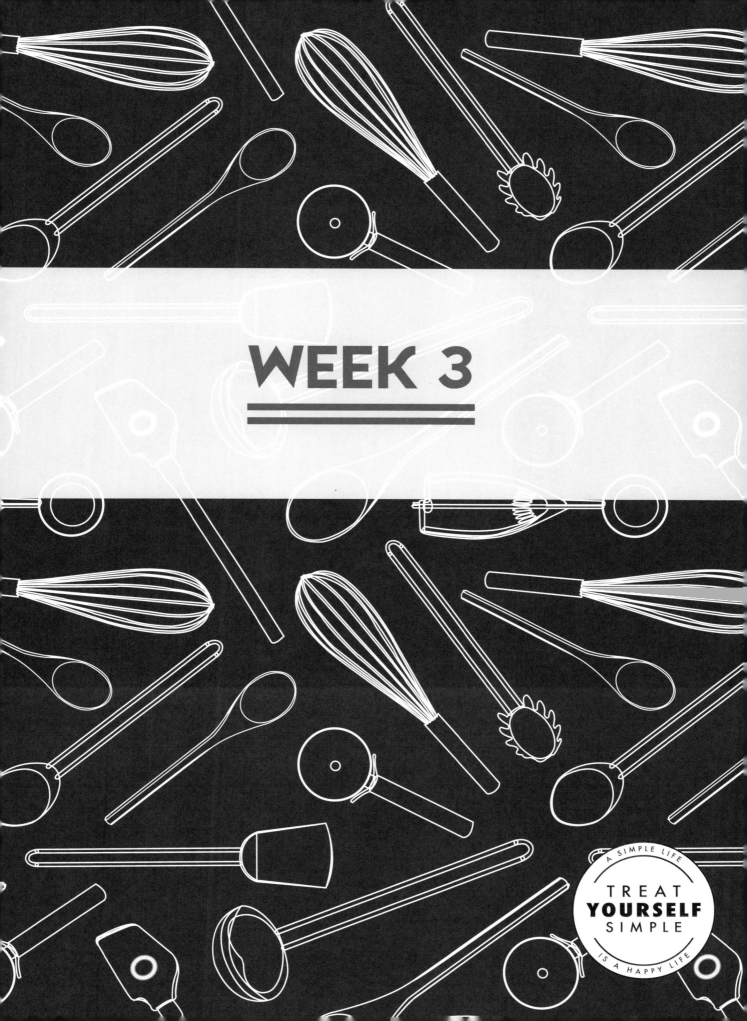

WEEK 3

WEEK 3 MENU PLAN

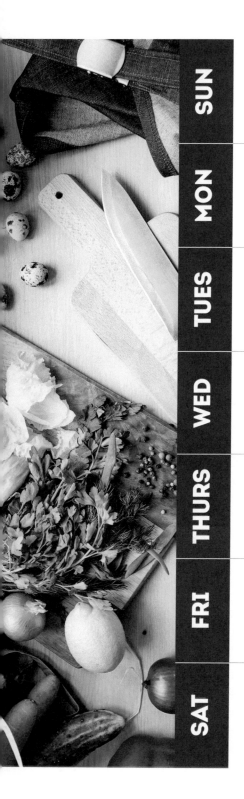

SUN

TERIYAKI SHRIMP

Quinoa
Orange Slices

MON

BBQ CHICKEN 2/1

Brussel Sprouts
Cinnamon Apples

TUES

TERIYAKI CHICKEN SALAD

Coleslaw
Banana Slices

WED

CHICKPEA SALAD SANDWICH

Sweet Potato Discs
Green Beans

THURS

BBQ CHICKEN PIZZA 2/1

Fresh Salad
Fresh Fruit Bowl

FRI

BALSAMIC PORK CHOPS

Coleslaw
Cinnamon Apples

SAT

BROCCOLI CHEESE SOUP

Fresh Salad
Pears

WEEK 3 GROCERY LIST

BY MEAL

TERIYAKI SHRIMP

2 T	Teriyaki Sauce
½ T	Sesame Seeds, toasted
½	Onion, red, small, fresh, cut into 4 wedges
¼ can	Pineapple, chunks, 14.5 oz can or ¼ C
12	Shrimp, large, peeled and deveined or 2 C Salad Shrimp

BBQ CHICKEN 2/1

1 T	Apple Cider Vinegar
4	Chicken Breasts, 4 oz each, 2 breasts for **BBQ Chicken Pizza 2**/1
¼ t	Garlic Powder
¼ C	Ketchup
¼ t	Kosher Salt
½ t	Mustard, ground
1 t	Olive Oil
½ t	Onion Powder
½ C	Onion, sweet, fresh, sliced
2 T	Maple Syrup
1 t	Worcestershire Sauce

TERIYAKI CHICKEN SALAD

2 T	Almonds, sliced
½ T	Apple Cider Vinegar
¼ C	Cabbage, red, shredded
½ C	Carrots, diced
2	Chicken Breasts, 4 oz each
¼ C	Edamame, shelled, frozen
2 t	Honey
2 C	Lettuce, Romaine, chopped
⅓ C	Mayonnaise (Dukes is my fav)
½ t	Mustard, yellow
1 T	Olive Oil
½ T	Sesame Seeds, toasted
½ C	Teriyaki Sauce

CHICKPEA SALAD SANDWICH

1 t	Apple Cider Vinegar
optional	Spinach, baby, fresh
dash	Black Pepper, ground
4 slices	Bread
optional	Carrots, fresh, shredded
¼ C	Onion, red, chopped
½ can	Chickpeas, 15 oz can, rinsed and drained
2 t	Dill, fresh, chopped
dash	Kosher Salt
2 T	Mayonnaise
2½ t	Mustard, yellow
⅛ t	Turmeric
optional	Sprouts, fresh
optional	Tomatoes, medium, fresh, sliced

BBQ CHICKEN PIZZA 2/1

½ C	BBQ Sauce from **BBQ Chicken 2/1**
⅔ C	Cheese, Gouda, shredded
⅔ C	Cheese, Mozzarella, shredded
2	Chicken Breasts, 4 oz each, from **BBQ Chicken 2/1**
optional	Cilantro, fresh
2 t	Olive Oil
¼ C	Onion, red, fresh, sliced thinly
1	Pizza Crust, canned

BALSAMIC PORK CHOPS

¼ C	Vinegar, Balsamic
¼ t	Black Pepper, ground
1½ C	Chicken Broth
1 T	Flour, all purpose
1½ t	Garlic, minced
⅓ t	Rosemary, fresh, chopped
¼ t	Kosher Salt
1½ T	Olive Oil
2	Pork Chops, 4 oz

BROCCOLI CHEESE SOUP

dash	Black Pepper, ground
1 C	Broccoli, frozen
2 T	Butter
½ C	Carrots, diced
optional	Pepper, red, crushed
¼ C	Cheese, Cheddar, shredded
2 T	Flour
1 C	Half & Half
1 t	Garlic, minced
dash	Kosher Salt
optional	Mustard, dried
½ T	Olive Oil
½ C	Onion, chopped
optional	Paprika, ground
1 C	Stock or Broth, Vegetable

WEEK 3 PREP

Mince 3 cloves Garlic ~ Balsamic Pork Chops, Broccoli Cheese Soup

Slice ½ small fresh Red Onion ~ BBQ Chicken 2/1

Cut ½ small fresh Red Onion into 4 wedges ~ Teriyaki Shrimp

Chop ½ small fresh Red Onion ~ Chickpea Salad Sandwich, BBQ Chicken Pizza 2/1

Slice 1½ small Sweet Onions ~ Broccoli Cheese Soup

Dice 1 C Carrots ~ Teriyaki Chicken Salad, Broccoli Cheese Soup

Shred ⅔ C Gouda Cheese ~ BBQ Chicken Pizza 2/1

Shred ⅔ Mozzarella Cheese ~ BBQ Chicken Pizza 2/1

Shred ½ C Cheddar Cheese ~ Broccoli Cheese Soup

WEEK 3 MAKE AHEAD

Prepare Marinade ~ BBQ Chicken 2/1

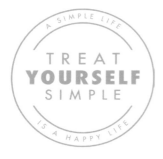

WEEK 3 RECIPES

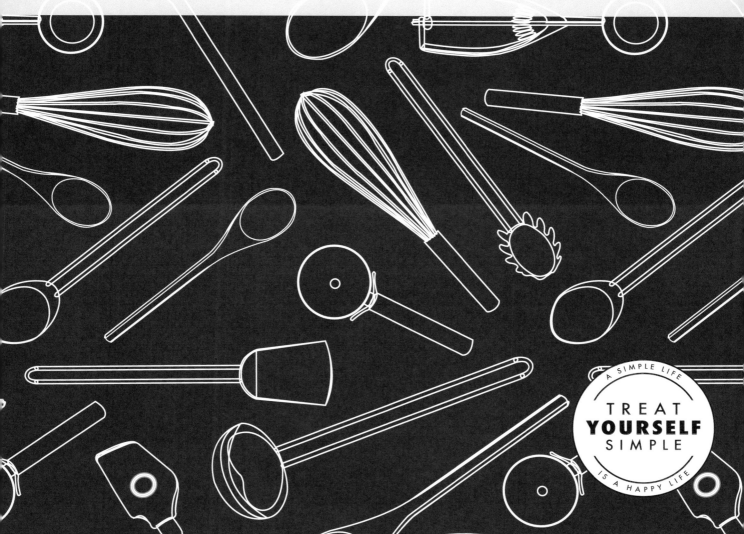

TREAT YOURSELF SIMPLE

A SIMPLE LIFE IS A HAPPY LIFE

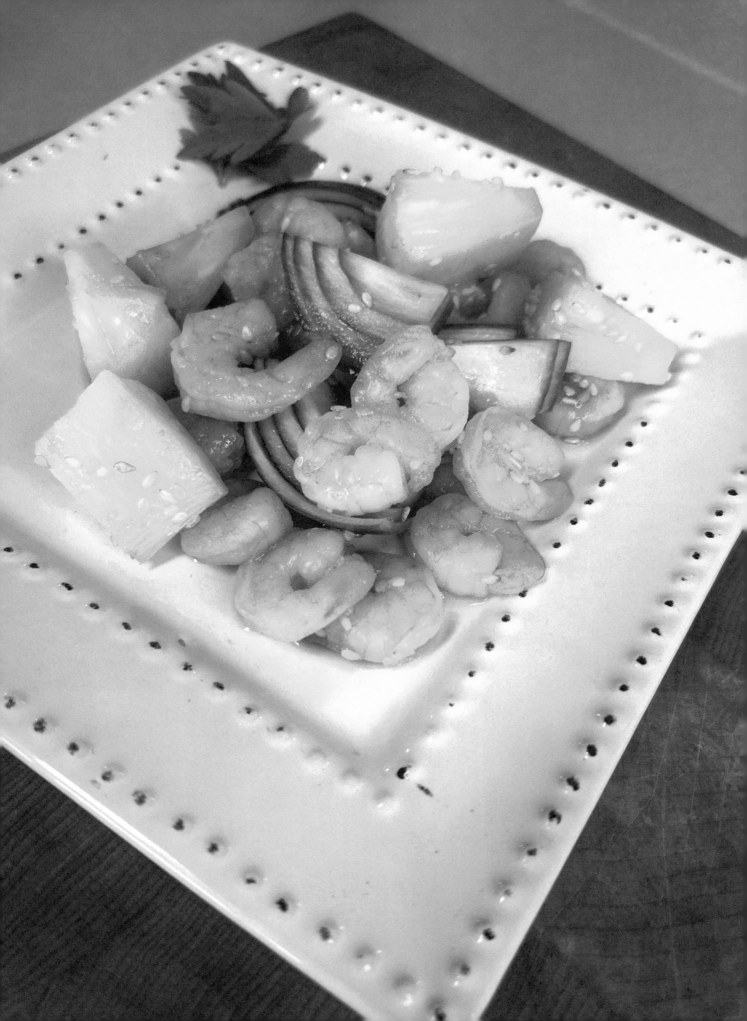

TERIYAKI SHRIMP   GRILL OR OVEN

Serving Size:	2 servings	Cook time:	16 minutes
Prep time:	15 minutes	Needed:	Aluminum foil, measuring cup or small bowl, baking sheet

DIRECTIONS

○ Preheat grill on high or oven at 350º F.

2 T ➤ Teriyaki Sauce
½ T ➤ Sesame Seeds, toasted

○ **Can make ahead. See Make Ahead Directions.** If not already prepared, combine the above ingredients in a measuring cup or small bowl; set aside.

½ ➤ Onion, red, small, fresh, cut into 4 wedges
¼ C ➤ Pineapple, chunks, 14.5 oz can or ¼ C
12 ➤ Shrimp, large, peeled and deveined or 2 C Salad Shrimp

○ Lay out two pieces of foil. Place shrimp mixture on one piece of foil.
Top with Teriyaki/Sesame Seed sauce, onion wedges, and pineapple chunks.
Place second piece of foil on top and seal pack.

GRILL
○ Place shrimp pack on grill.

OVEN
○ Place on baking sheet.

○ Grill or bake about 10 minutes until shrimp is pink and reaches 165º F.

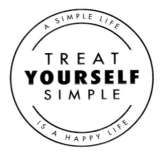

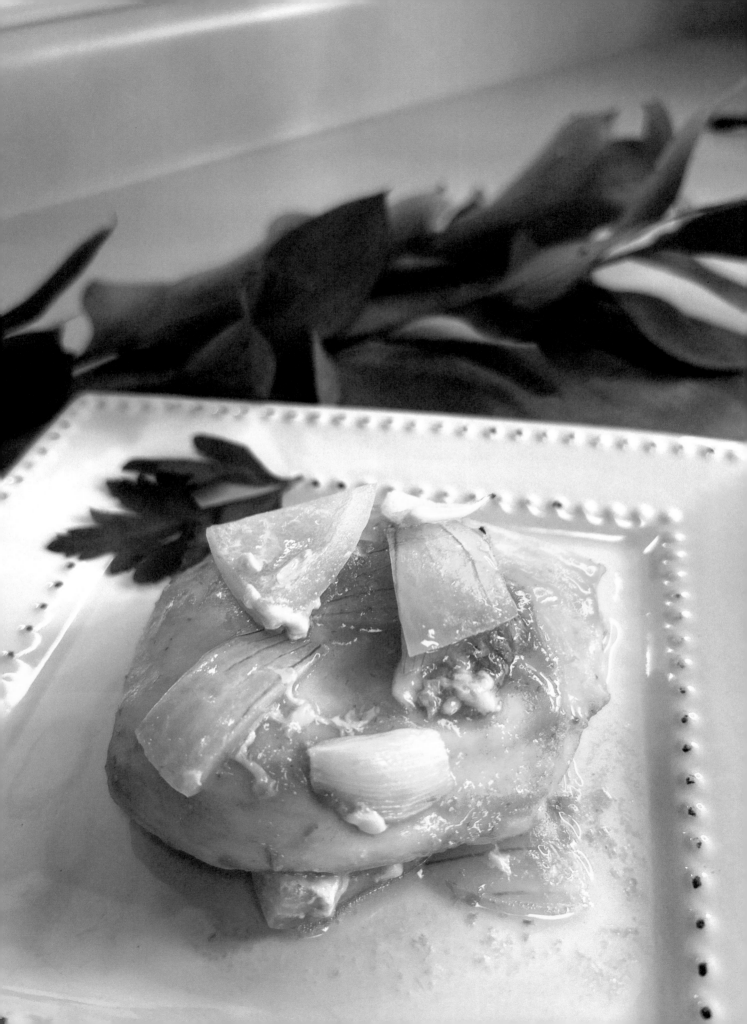

BBQ CHICKEN 2/1 OVEN

Please note: Makes Chicken for BBQ Chicken Pizza 2/1

Serving Size:	2 servings	Cook time:	40 minutes
Prep time:	1 hour 10 minutes	Needed:	Medium mixing bowl, zip top bag, baking sheet, aluminum foil, cooking spray, spatula

DIRECTIONS

1 T ➤ Apple Cider Vinegar
4 ➤ Chicken Breasts, 4 oz each
¼ t ➤ Garlic Powder
¼ C ➤ Ketchup
¼ t ➤ Kosher Salt
2 T ➤ Maple Syrup
½ t ➤ Mustard, ground
½ t ➤ Onion Powder
1 t ➤ Worcestershire Sauce

MARINADE

○ **Can make ahead. See Make Ahead Directions.** If not already prepared, combine the above ingredients in a medium mixing bowl (minus the chicken); reserve ½ C of sauce for **BBQ Chicken Pizza.** Add chicken and remaining barbeque sauce to zip top bag or sealed container. Refrigerate for at least 1 hour and up to overnight.

1 t ➤ Olive Oil
½ C ➤ Onion, sweet, fresh, sliced

○ Preheat oven to 425° F. Line, a baking sheet, with aluminum foil and coat with cooking spray. Place, on baking sheet, onions; drizzle with oil; toss to coat. Place chicken on top of onions; bake until golden and internal temperature reaches 165° F (15 minutes). Remove from heat; Serve remaining 2 chicken breasts warm.

NOTE: *Remove half of the chicken breasts for* **BBQ Chicken Pizza 2/1.** *Set aside, cool, and store in an airtight container. Refrigerate for 7–10 days.*

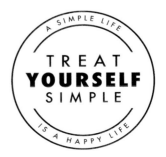

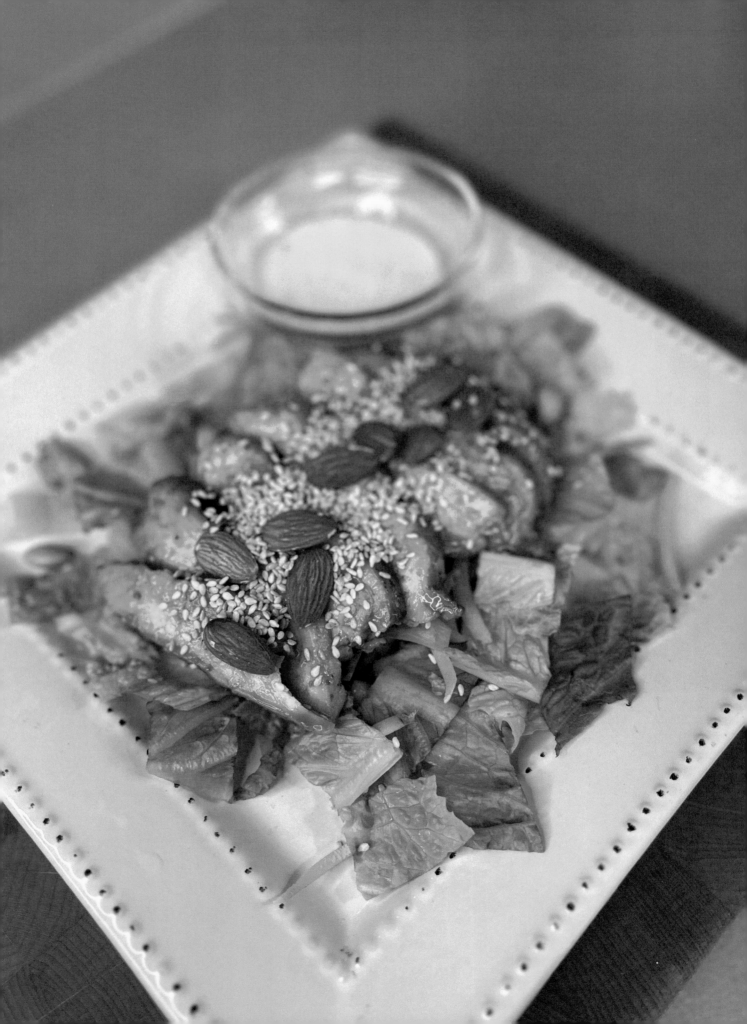

TERIYAKI CHICKEN SALAD   OVEN

Serving Size:	2 servings	Cook time:	15 minutes
Prep time:	30 minutes	Needed:	Zip top bag or sealed container, casserole dish, measuring cup, medium mixing bowl, spatula

DIRECTIONS

2 ➤ Chicken Breasts, 4 oz each
½ C ➤ Teriyaki Sauce

○ Place chicken in zip top bag or sealed container. Add teriyaki sauce. Rub teriyaki sauces over the chicken. Place into refrigerator for 30 minutes.

WHEN READY TO COOK

○ Preheat oven to 400° F. Coat a casserole dish with 1 T olive oil; add chicken and sauce to casserole dish; bake for 10–12 minutes until internal temperature reaches 165° F. Remove from heat; set aside.

½ T ➤ Apple Cider Vinegar
2 t ➤ Honey
⅓ C ➤ Mayonnaise
½ t ➤ Mustard, yellow
1 T ➤ Olive Oil

○ Add the above ingredients in a measuring cup or small bowl; whisk together until well blended; refrigerate until ready to serve.

¼ C ➤ Cabbage, red, shredded
½ C ➤ Carrots, diced
¼ C ➤ Edamame, shelled, frozen
2 C ➤ Lettuce, Romaine, chopped

○ Add the above ingredients in a medium mixing bowl; toss together. Set aside.

2 T ➤ Almonds, sliced
½ T ➤ Sesame Seeds, toasted

○ Divide the salad mixture onto two plates; slice each chicken breast into strips; divide on top of salad mixture.

○ Sprinkle sliced almonds and sesame seeds over chicken and salad mixture. Drizzle with prepared dressing. Serve immediately.

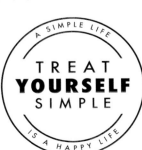

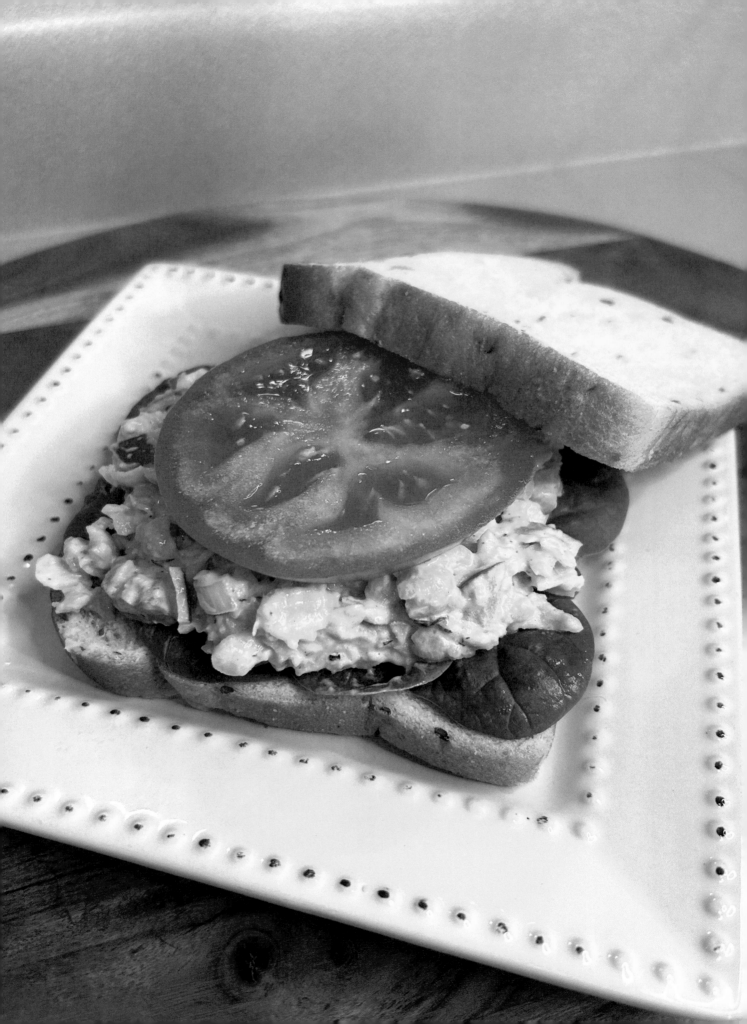

CHICKPEA SALAD SANDWICH NO COOK

Serving Size:	2 servings	Cook time:	No cooking required
Prep time:	10 minutes	Needed:	Medium mixing bowl, spoon

DIRECTIONS

1 t ➤ Apple Cider Vinegar
dash ➤ Black Pepper, ground
½ can ➤ Chickpeas, 15 oz can, rinsed and drained
2 t ➤ Dill, fresh, chopped
dash ➤ Kosher Salt
2 T ➤ Mayonnaise
2 ½ t ➤ Mustard, yellow
¼ C ➤ Onion, red, chopped
⅛ t ➤ Turmeric, ground

○ Add chickpeas to a medium mixing bowl; mash.
Then, add the rest of the above ingredients and mix well.

4 slices ➤ Bread
optional ➤ Carrots, fresh, shredded
optional ➤ Spinach, baby, fresh
optional ➤ Sprouts, fresh
optional ➤ Tomatoes, medium, fresh, sliced

○ Place one bread slice each on two plates.
Spread with half of the above mixture; add the optional above ingredients;
top sandwich with a slice of bread. Serve immediately.

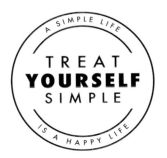

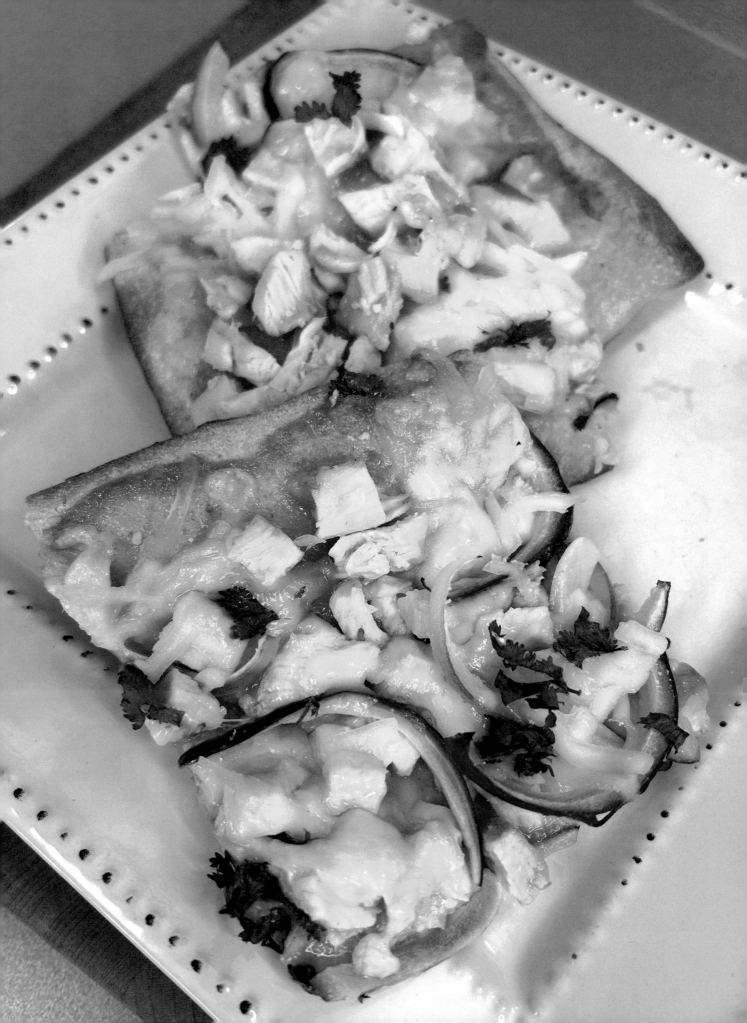

BBQ CHICKEN PIZZA 2/1   OVEN

Please note: Chicken was prepared from BBQ Chicken 2/1

Serving Size:	2 servings	Cook time:	15 minutes
Prep time:	15 minutes	Needed:	Baking sheet, spatula, spoon

DIRECTIONS

1 ➤ Pizza Crust, canned

○ Prepare pizza crust according to package instructions. Remove from heat.

2 t ➤ Olive Oil
½ C ➤ BBQ Sauce from **BBQ Chicken 2/1**
2 ➤ Chicken Breasts, 4 oz each, shredded, from **BBQ Chicken 2/1**
⅔ C ➤ Cheese, Mozzarella, shredded
⅔ C ➤ Cheese, Gouda, shredded
¼ C ➤ Onion, red, fresh, sliced thinly
optional ➤ Cilantro, fresh, chopped

○ Spread olive oil on cooked pizza crust; then BBQ sauce;
layer shredded chicken and onions; sprinkle cheese to cover pizza crust;
garnish with optional ingredient.

○ Bake pizza until cheese is melted, about 10 minutes.
Remove from heat and let cool for 5 minutes; slice pizza. Serve warm.

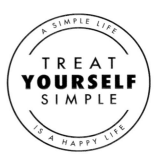

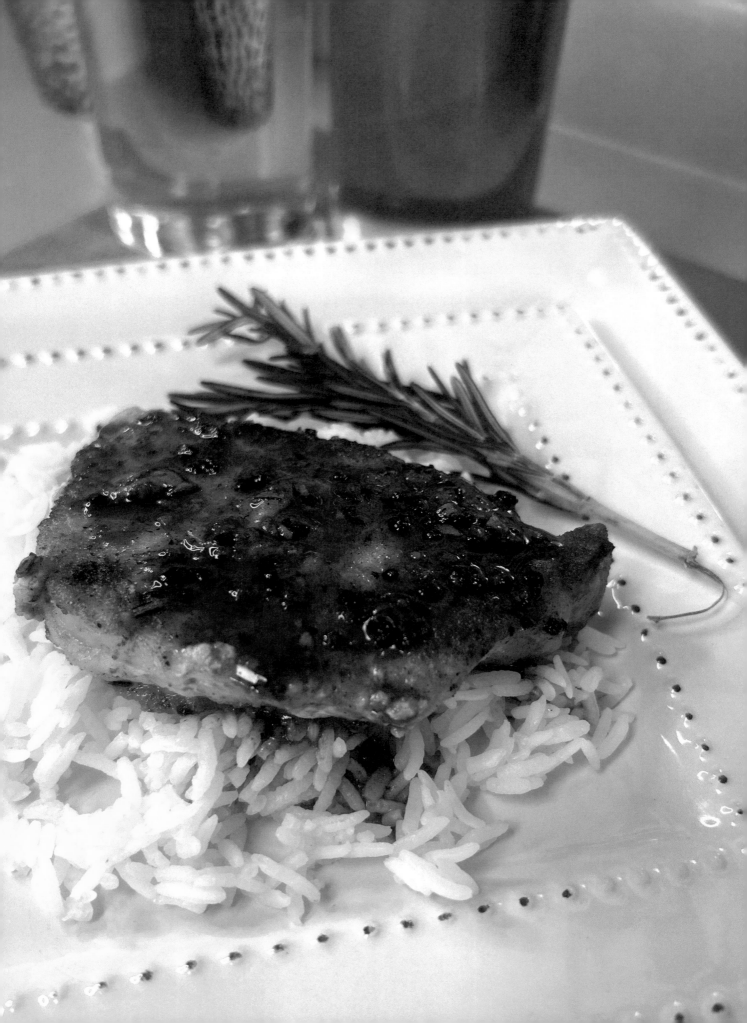

BALSAMIC PORK CHOPS STOVE

Serving Size:	2 servings	Cook time:	25 minutes
Prep time:	10 minutes	Needed:	Shallow casserole dish, skillet, spatula

DIRECTIONS

1 T ➤ Flour, all purpose
⅓ t ➤ Rosemary, fresh, chopped
¼ t ➤ Kosher Salt
¼ t ➤ Black Pepper, ground

○ Combine the above ingredients in a shallow casserole dish.

2 ➤ Pork Chops, 4 oz

○ Dredge above ingredient in flour mixture until both sides are coated.

1 ½ T ➤ Olive Oil

○ Add above ingredient to skillet over medium-high heat.

1 ½ t ➤ Garlic, minced

○ Add above ingredient to skillet. Sauté 1 minute. Add pork chops to skillet, cooking for about 4 minutes on each side or until golden.
Remove pork chops. Place on plate.

1 ½ C ➤ Chicken Broth
¼ C ➤ Vinegar, Balsamic

○ Add above ingredients to skillet, stirring to loosen particles from bottom of skillet. Cook about 6 minutes or until liquid is reduced by half.
Add pork chops, cook 5 minutes or until done to temp.
Garnish with rosemary sprigs. Serve warm.

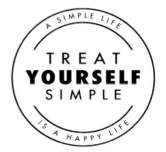

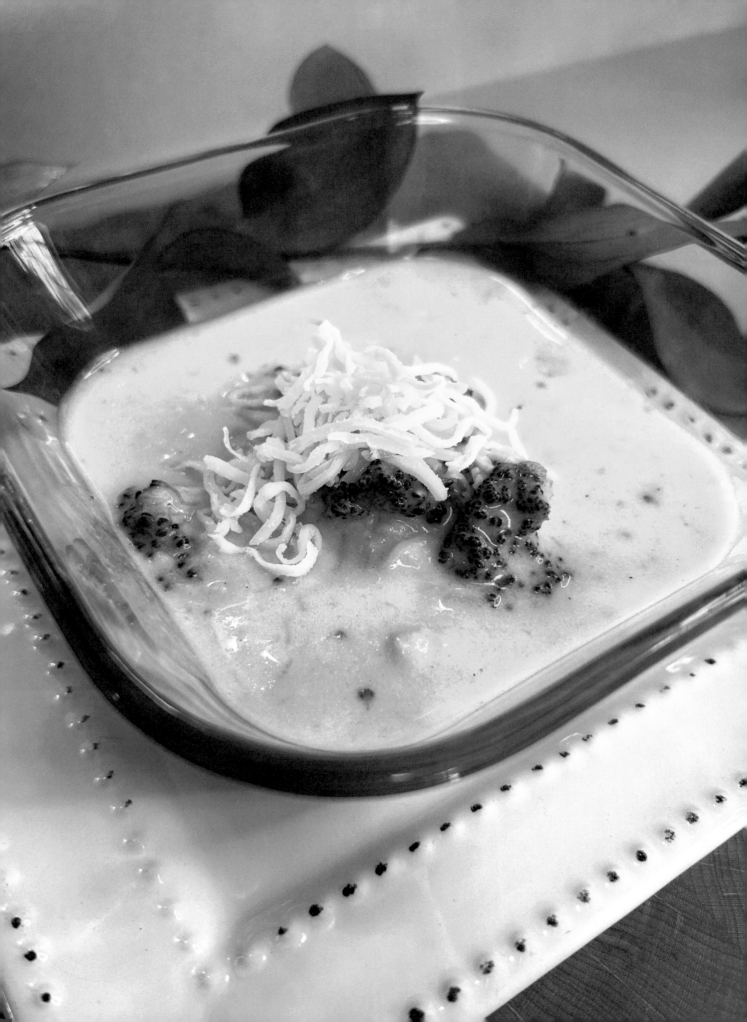

BROCCOLI CHEESE SOUP STOVE

Serving Size:	2 servings	Cook time:	45 minutes
Prep time:	15 minutes	Needed:	Medium saucepan, heat-safe spoon

DIRECTIONS

½ T ➤ Olive Oil
½ C ➤ Onion, chopped
1 t ➤ Garlic, minced

○ Coat skillet with olive oil over medium heat. Add above ingredients.
Cook for about 3 minutes until the onion is translucent and barely browned.
Stir intermittently.

2 T ➤ Flour
2 T ➤ Butter

○ Add the above ingredients. Cook over medium heat for 1–2 minutes,
stirring constantly, until the flour is thickened.

1 C ➤ Stock or Broth, Vegetable
1 C ➤ Half & Half

○ Add above ingredients, stirring constantly. Simmer over low heat
for about 15 minutes or until reduced and thickened. Stir intermittently
to reincorporate the skin that inevitably forms. This is normal.

1 C ➤ Broccoli, frozen
½ C ➤ Carrots, diced
dash ➤ Paprika, ground
dash ➤ Mustard, dried
dash ➤ Pepper, red, crushed
dash ➤ Kosher Salt
dash ➤ Black Pepper, ground

○ Add above ingredients to pan. Simmer for 10 minutes.
Stir intermittently to reincorporate the "skin" that forms. This is normal.

¼ C ➤ Cheese, Cheddar, shredded

○ Stir in cheese until fully melted, about 1 minute.
Transfer to bowls, garnishing with additional cheese.
Serve warm.

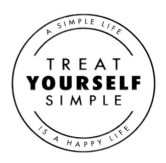

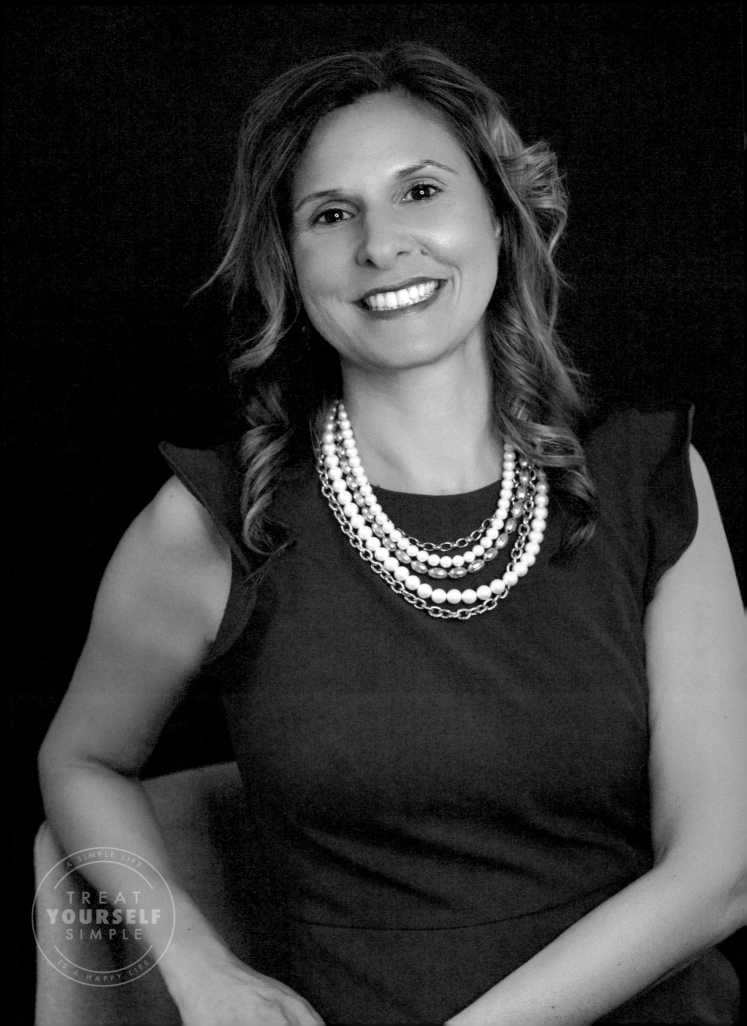

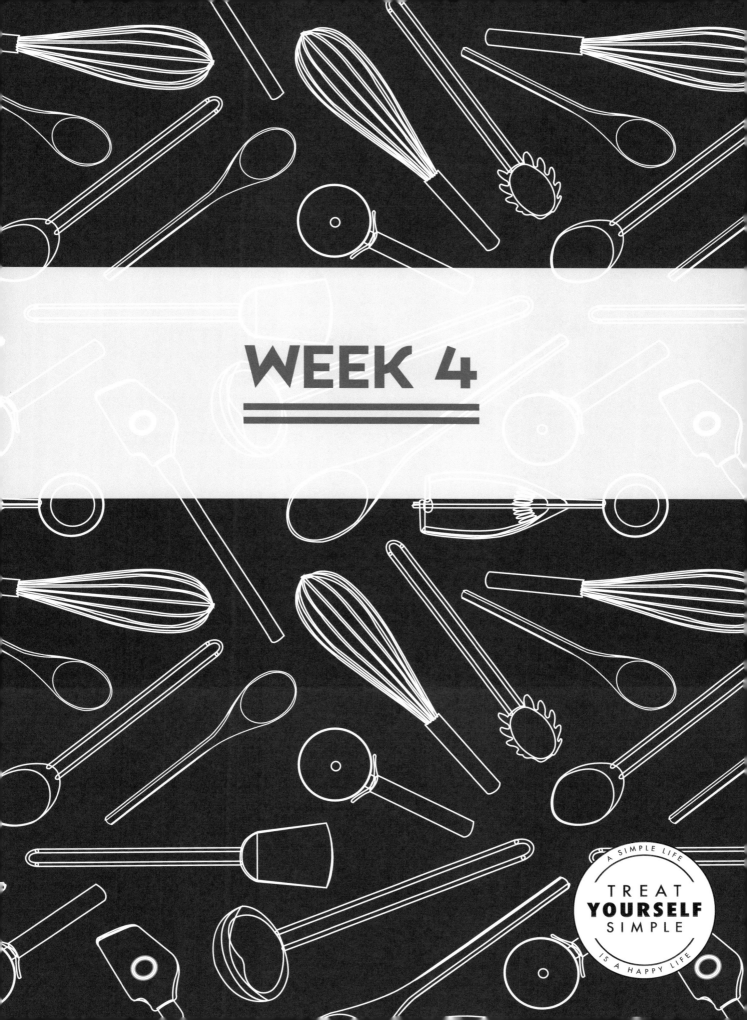

WEEK 4

WEEK 4 MENU PLAN

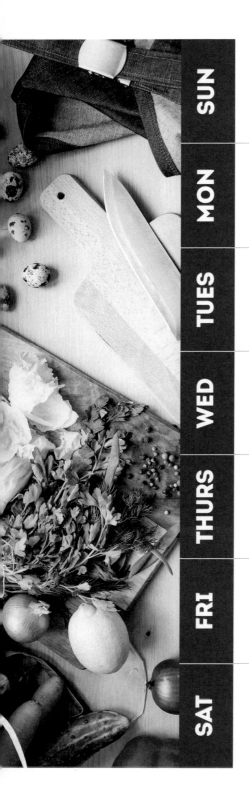

SUN

BISTRO FALL SALAD

Baguette
Orange Slices

MON

RANCHERO SUPPER 2/1

Broccoli
Cinnamon Apples

TUES

GARLIC SHRIMP & TOMATO PASTA

Fresh Salad
Pears

WED

SLOPPY JOES 2/1

Coleslaw
Green Beans

THURS

CHICKEN NOODLE SOUP

Fresh Salad
Fresh Fruit Bowl

FRI

QUICK TUNA MELT

Sweet Potato Discs
Cinnamon Apples

SAT

FETA SHRIMP TACOS

Fresh Salad
Pears

WEEK 4 GROCERY LIST

BY MEAL

BISTRO FALL SALAD

6 T	Walnuts, chopped
½ T	Butter
½ T	Honey
2 T	Olive Oil
2 T	Vinegar, Balsamic
1½ T	Maple Syrup
½ t	Mustard, Dijon
⅛ t	Thyme, dried
dash	Kosher Salt
dash	Black Pepper, ground
1	Apple, medium, cored and sliced
¼ C	Cheese, Feta, crumbled
	Cranberries, dried
3 C	Lettuce, Romaine, chopped

RANCHERO SUPPER 2/1

½ can	Baked Beans, 14 oz can
¼ C	BBQ Sauce
1 lb	Beef, ground, ½ for **Sloppy Joes 2/1**
¾ C	Cheese, Cheddar, shredded
2 T	Ketchup
1 T	Mustard, yellow
optional	Onion, green, fresh, sliced
optional	Sour Cream
2 C	Tortilla Chips
½ C	Corn, frozen

GARLIC SHRIMP & TOMATO PASTA

¼ C	Apple Juice
¼ t	Pepper, red, crushed
1½ t	Garlic, minced
1½ T	Parsley, fresh, chopped
dash	Kosher Salt
½ T	Lemon Juice
1 T + ½ T	Olive Oil
2 T	Onion, sweet, fresh, chopped
¼ t	Oregano, dried
4 oz	Pasta, spaghetti noodles
12	Shrimp, large, peeled, tail off or 2 C Salad Shrimp
1 C	Tomatoes, cherry, fresh, halved
garnish	Cheese, Parmesan, shredded

SLOPPY JOES 2/1

3 T	BBQ Sauce, Honey-style
2	Buns, Hamburger, lightly toasted
optional	Cheese, Colby Jack, slices
½ lb	Beef, ground, from **Ranchero Supper 2/1**
3 T	Ketchup
1 t	Mustard, yellow
optional	Pickles
1 T	Honey

CHICKEN NOODLE SOUP

1½ T	Olive Oil
2	Chicken Breasts, 4 oz each, cut into bite-sized pieces
2 t	Garlic, minced
1	Onion, sweet, chopped
2 stalks	Celery, chopped
1	Carrot, chopped
⅓ C	Bell Peppers, any color, diced
½ t	Thyme, fresh, chopped
½ t	Parsley, fresh, chopped
½ t	Oregano, fresh, chopped
½ t	Kosher Salt
¼ t	Black Pepper, ground
2 t	Better than Bouillon, Chicken base or 2 cubes Chicken Bouillon
1 C	Pasta, (cavatapppi, elbows, spirals, etc.)

QUICK TUNA MELT

dash	Black Pepper, ground
4 slices	Bread
1 T	Butter
½ stalk	Celery, fresh, chopped
2	Cheese, Cheddar, slices
dash	Pepper, red, crushed
1 T	Parsley, fresh, chopped
dash	Kosher Salt
½ T	Lemon Juice
2½ T	Mayonnaise
2 T	Onion, sweet, fresh, chopped
1 T	Pickles, Dill, chopped
2	Tomato, medium, fresh, slices
1 can	Tuna, 5 oz can

FETA SHRIMP TACOS

BY MEAL

optional	Avocado, fresh, sliced
dash	Black Pepper, ground
4	Tortilla Shells, 6–8", Flour or Corn
2 T	Mayonnaise
2 T	Onion, sweet, fresh, chopped
12	Shrimp, large, peeled and deveined or 2 C Salad Shrimp
¼ C	Cheese, Feta, crumbled
½ T	Apple Cider Vinegar
½ T	Mustard
½ T	Olive Oil
½ T	Taco Seasoning
½	Banana Pepper, fresh, chopped or if from jar, ¼ C
1 C	Cabbage, red or green, fresh, shredded

WEEK 4 PREP

Mince 4 Garlic cloves ~ Garlic Shrimp & Tomato Pasta, Chicken Noodle Soup,

Dice Chicken Breast into bite-sized pieces ~ Chicken Noodle Soup

Chop 1¾ Sweet Onions ~ Garlic Shrimp & Tomato Pasta, Chicken Noodle Soup, Quick Tuna Melt, Feta Shrimp Tacos

Chop 1 Carrot ~ Chicken Noodle Soup

Chop 3 stalks Celery ~ Chicken Noodle Soup, Quick Tuna Melt

Shred 1 C Red Cabbage ~ Feta Shrimp Tacos

Shred ¾ C Cheddar Cheese ~ Ranchero Supper 2/1

WEEK 4 MAKE AHEAD

Make Dressing ~ Bistro Fall Salad

Prepare Taco Seasoning ~ Feta Shrimp Tacos

NOTES

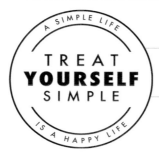

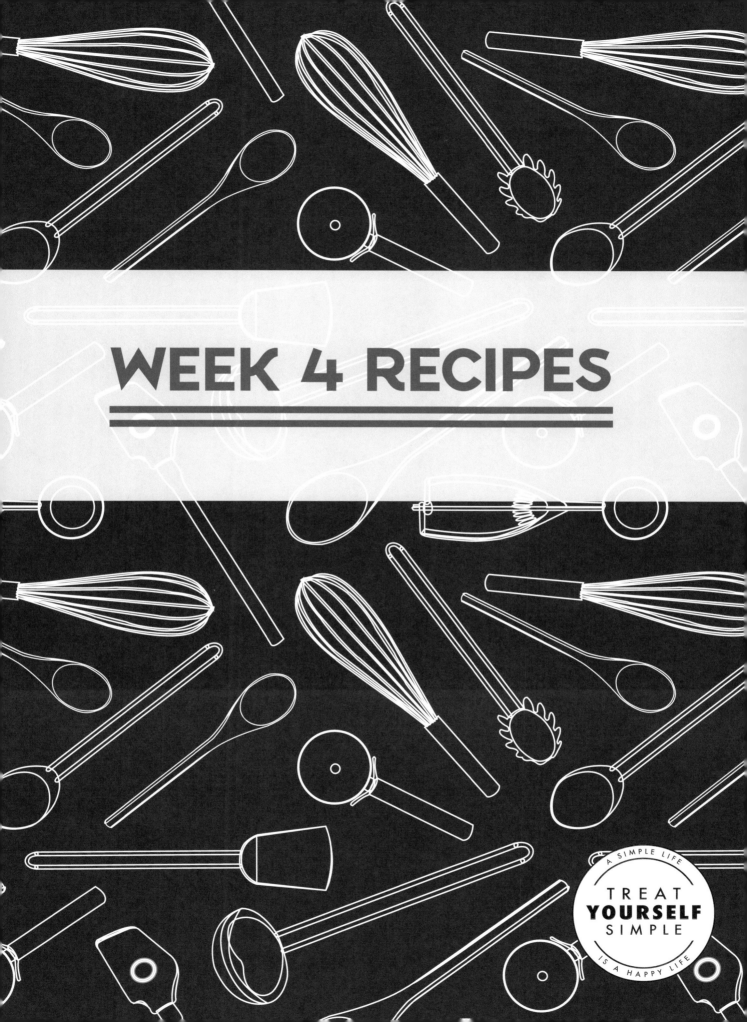

WEEK 4 RECIPES

TREAT **YOURSELF** SIMPLE

A SIMPLE LIFE

IS A HAPPY LIFE

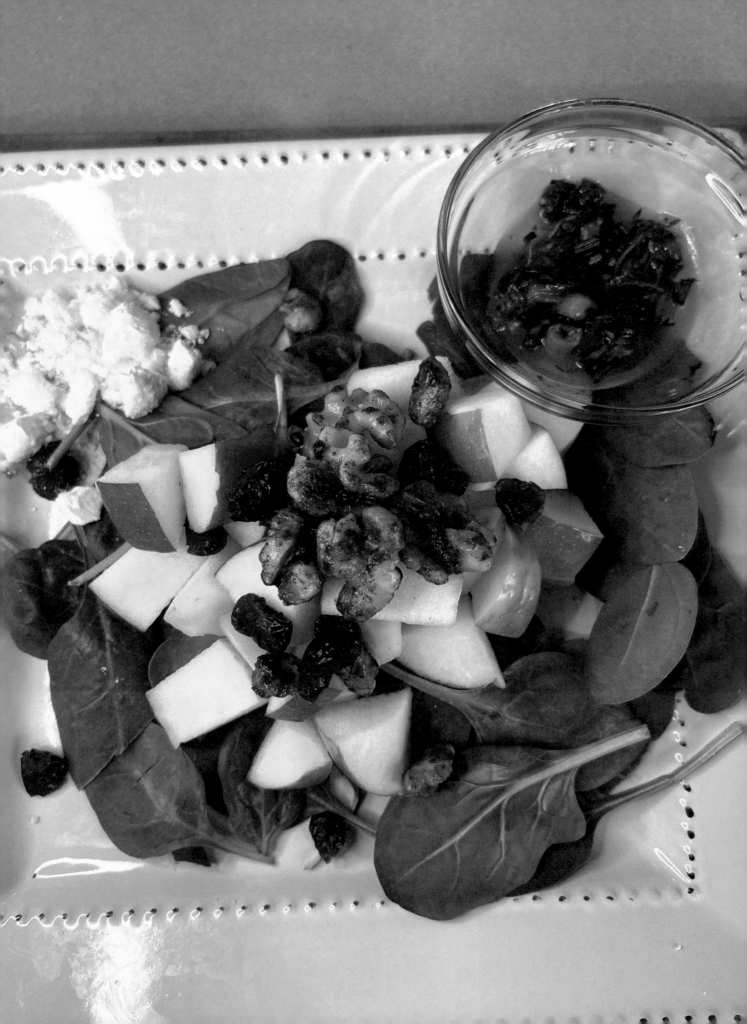

BISTRO FALL SALAD   OVEN

Serving Size:	2 servings	Cook time:	10 minutes
Prep time:	10 minutes	Needed:	Jar, skillet, large salad bowl, spatula, spoon

DIRECTIONS

6 T ➤ Walnuts, chopped
½ T ➤ Butter
½ T ➤ Honey

○ **To make the candied walnuts:** In a medium skillet over high heat, sauté the above ingredients until the walnuts are coated, beginning to turn golden brown and fragrant (about 5 minutes). Remove from heat and cool.

2 T ➤ Olive Oil
2 T ➤ Vinegar, Balsamic
1½ T ➤ Maple Syrup
½ t ➤ Mustard, Dijon
⅛ t ➤ Thyme, dried
dash ➤ Kosher Salt
dash ➤ Black Pepper, ground

DRESSING

○ **Can make ahead. See Make Ahead Directions.** If not already prepared, combine the above ingredients in a jar with a tight fitting lid. Shake the dressing until smooth and season with salt & pepper to taste. Set in fridge until ready to use.

1 ➤ Apple, medium, cored and sliced
¼ C ➤ Cheese, Feta, crumbled
➤ Cranberries, dried

○ Combine the above ingredients in a large bowl. Add the walnuts to the salad mixture.

3 C ➤ Lettuce, Romaine, chopped

○ Divide lettuce onto two plates. Divide apple mixture over lettuce.

○ Drizzle dressing over apple mixture on lettuce. Enjoy cold.

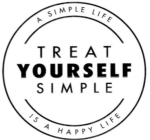

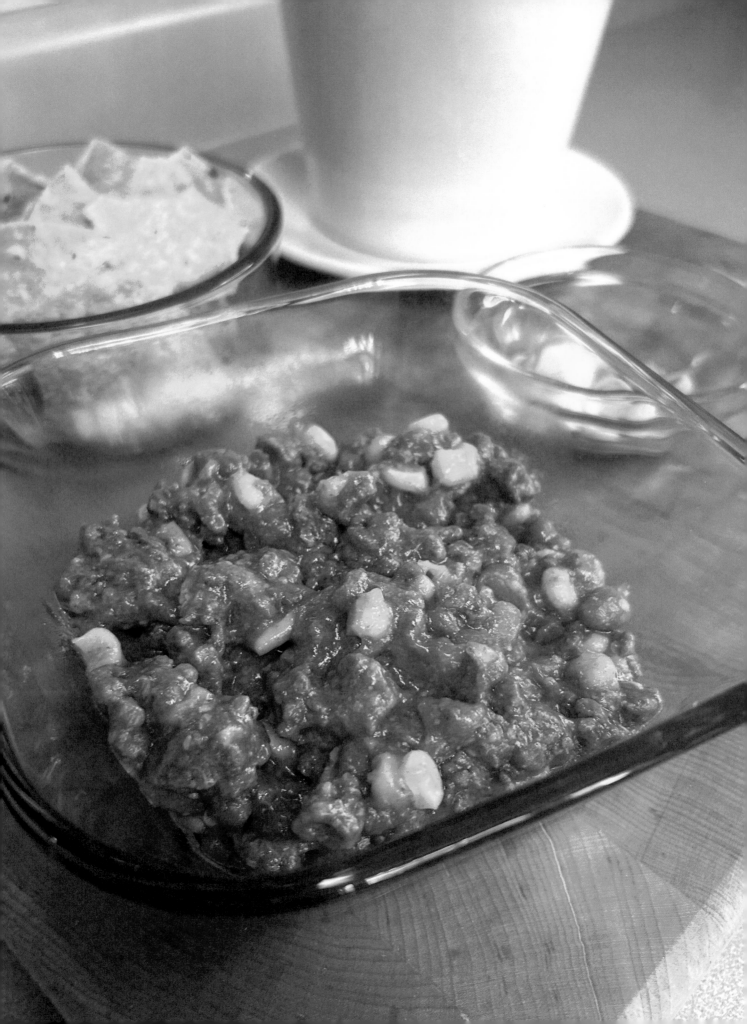

RANCHERO SUPPER 2/1 STOVE

Please note: Makes Ground Beef for Sloppy Joes 2/1

Serving Size:	2 servings	Cook time:	15 minutes
Prep time:	15 minutes	Needed:	Large skillet, heat-safe spoon

DIRECTIONS

1 lb ➤ Beef, ground, half for **Sloppy Joes 2/1**
½ can ➤ Baked Beans, 14 oz can
¼ C ➤ BBQ Sauce
¾ C ➤ Cheese, Cheddar, shredded
2 T ➤ Ketchup
1 T ➤ Mustard, Yellow\
½ C ➤ Corn, frozen

○ Add beef in skillet over medium heat; cook for 8–10 minutes, breaking meat apart into small pieces until no longer pink; drain, if needed; place beef back in skillet.

○ Add the rest of the ingredients in the skillet, sprinkling the cheese on last; mix well; cook for 5–8 minutes, stirring occasionally, until heated through and cheese has melted; set aside.

2 C ➤ Tortilla Chips
optional ➤ Onion, green, fresh, sliced
optional ➤ Sour Cream

○ Divide tortilla chips, half of the beef mixture, and optional ingredients. Serve warm.

NOTE: *Remove half of the ground beef mixture for* **Sloppy Joes 2/1.** *Set aside, cool, and store in an airtight container. Refrigerate for 7–10 days.*

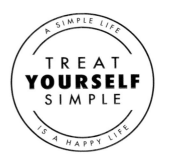

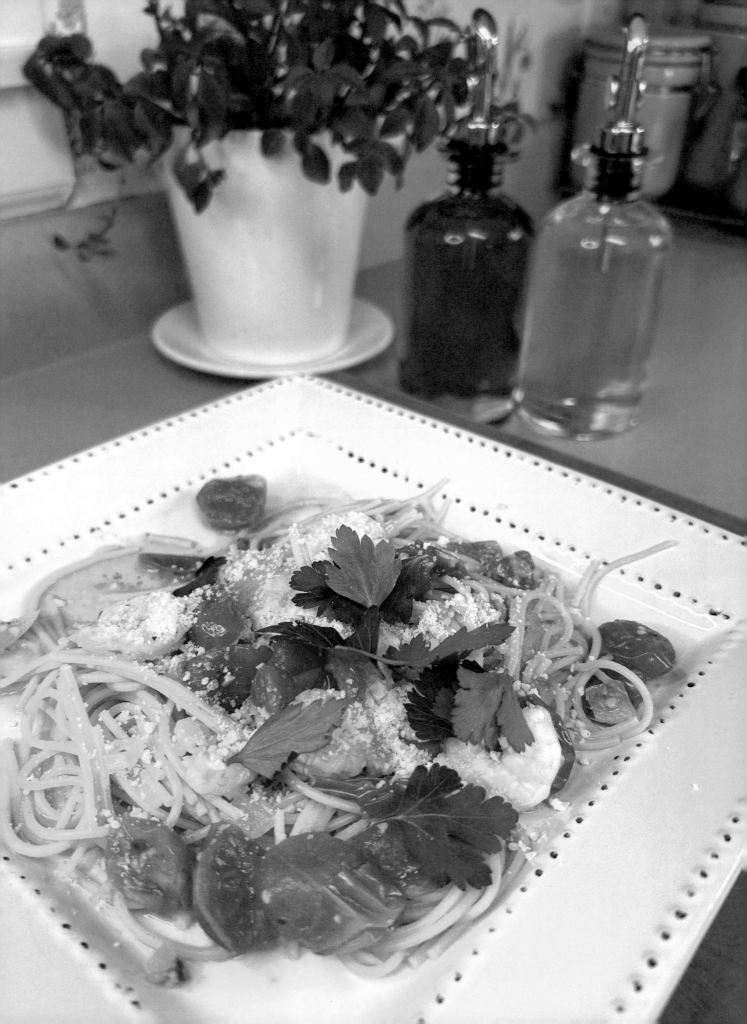

GARLIC SHRIMP & TOMATO PASTA STOVE

Serving Size:	2 servings	Cook time:	10 minutes
Prep time:	15 minutes	Needed:	Large skillet, medium saucepan, colander, heat-safe spoon

DIRECTIONS

4 oz ➤ Pasta, spaghetti noodles

○ Prepare pasta according to package instructions. Drain and set aside.

½ T ➤ Olive Oil
12 ➤ Shrimp, large, peeled and deveined, tail off or 2 C Salad Shrimp
dash ➤ Kosher Salt

○ Coat skillet with olive oil over medium heat. Add the above ingredients; cook, flipping often, until internal temperature reaches 145° F. Remove from heat; transfer to a plate and set aside.

1 T ➤ Olive Oil
2 T ➤ Onion, sweet, fresh, chopped
1½ t ➤ Garlic, minced
¼ C ➤ Apple Juice
¼ t ➤ Pepper, red, crushed
½ T ➤ Lemon Juice
¼ t ➤ Oregano, dried
1 C ➤ Tomatoes, cherry, fresh, halved

○ Coat skillet with olive oil over medium heat. Add onion and garlic, cooking about 3 minutes, until onions are translucent.
Add rest of above ingredients; bring to a simmer, stirring often, for about 3–5 minutes. Turn heat off; set aside.

garnish ➤ Cheese, Parmesan, shredded
1½ T ➤ Parsley, fresh, chopped

○ Divide pasta on two plates; divide sauce over pasta on each plate; divide shrimp onto each of the plates; sprinkle with Parmesan cheese and parsley. Serve warm.

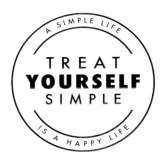

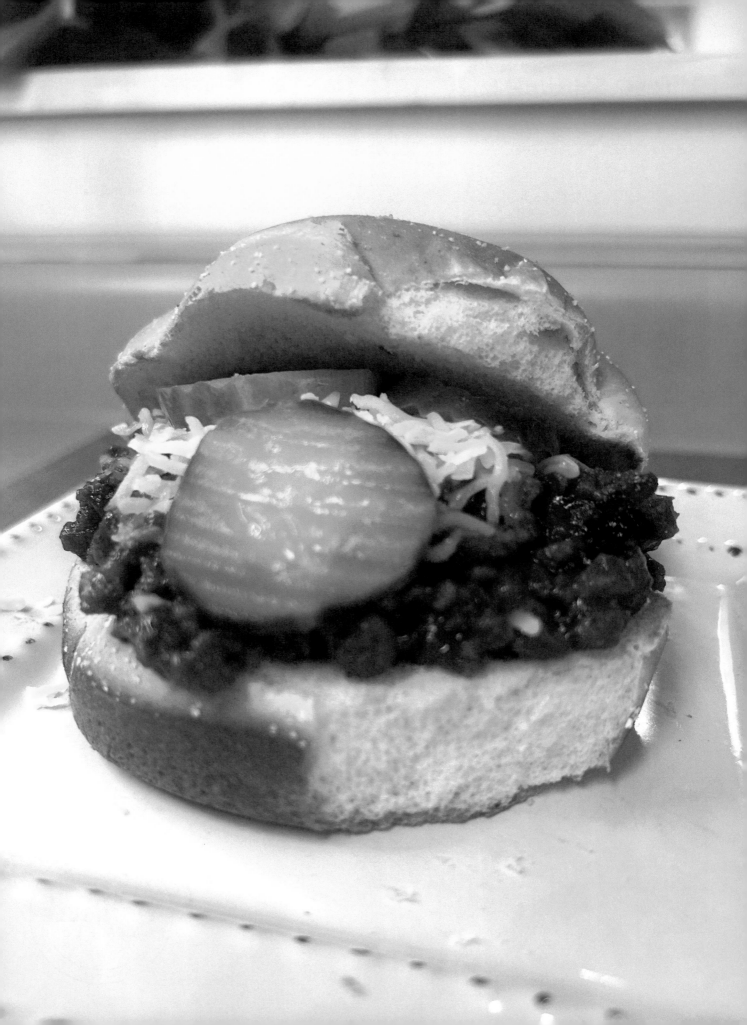

SLOPPY JOES 2/1 STOVE

Please note: Ground Beef was prepared from Ranchero Supper 2/1

Serving Size:	2 servings	Cook time:	20 minutes
Prep time:	5 minutes	Needed:	Large skillet, heat-safe spoon

DIRECTIONS

½ lb ➤ Beef, ground, from **Ranchero Supper 2/1**
3 T ➤ BBQ Sauce, Honey-style
3 T ➤ Ketchup
1 t ➤ Mustard, yellow
1 T ➤ Honey

○ Add the above ingredients into skillet; mix thoroughly until all meat is completely covered; Heat on medium for 3–5 minutes, stirring occasionally, until desired warmth is reached.

2 ➤ Buns, Hamburger, lightly toasted
optional ➤ Cheese, Colby Jack, slices
optional ➤ Pickles

○ Divide, on two plates, bottom of bun, ground beef mixture, optional ingredients, and top of bun. Serve warm.

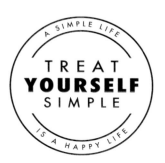

A SIMPLE LIFE
TREAT
YOURSELF
SIMPLE
IS A HAPPY LIFE

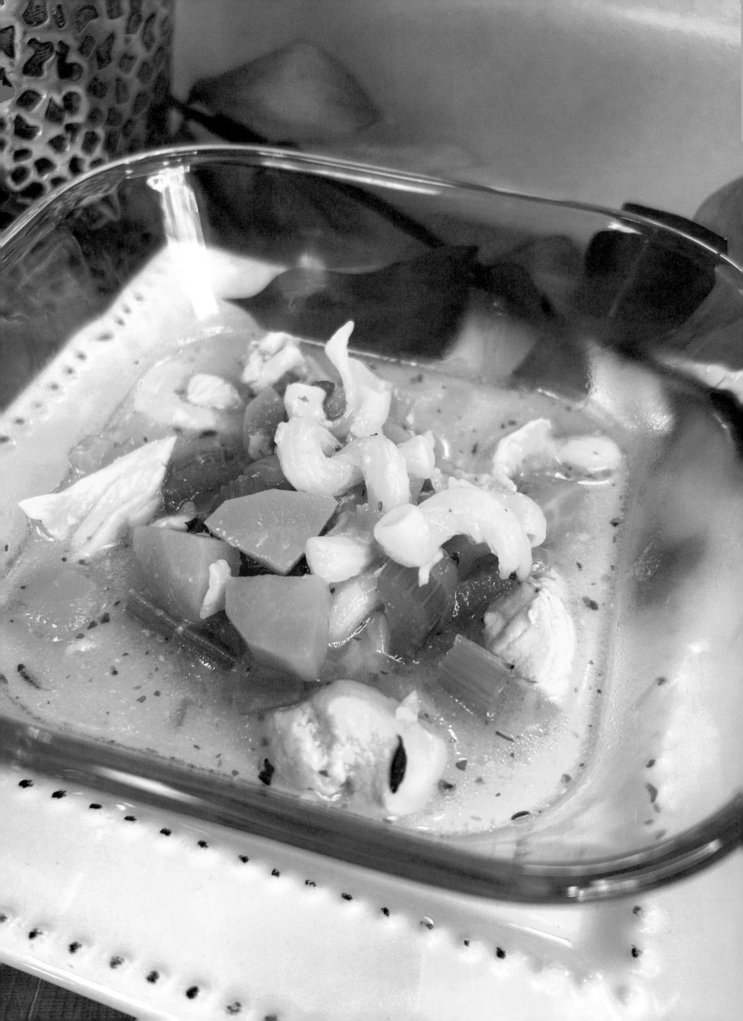

CHICKEN NOODLE SOUP STOVE

Serving Size:	2 servings	Cook time:	30 minutes
Prep time:	10 minutes	Needed:	Medium saucepan, heat-safe spoon

DIRECTIONS

1½ T ➤ Olive Oil
2 ➤ Chicken Breasts, 4 oz each, cut into bite-sized pieces

○ Coat skillet with olive oil over medium heat.
Add chicken, cooking for 12 minutes.

2 t ➤ Garlic, minced
1 ➤ Onion, sweet, chopped
2 stalks ➤ Celery, chopped
1 ➤ Carrot, chopped
⅓ C ➤ Bell Peppers, any color, diced
½ t ➤ Thyme, fresh, chopped
½ t ➤ Parsley, fresh, chopped
½ t ➤ Oregano, fresh, chopped
½ t ➤ Kosher Salt
¼ t ➤ Black Pepper, ground
2 t ➤ Better than Bouillon, Chicken base or 2 cubes Chicken Boullion)
1 C ➤ Pasta, (cavatapppi, elbows, spirals, etc.)

○ Stir in above ingredients. Cover and cook for 20 minutes.

○ Divide between two bowls. Serve immediately.

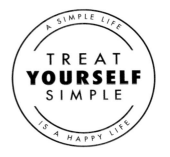

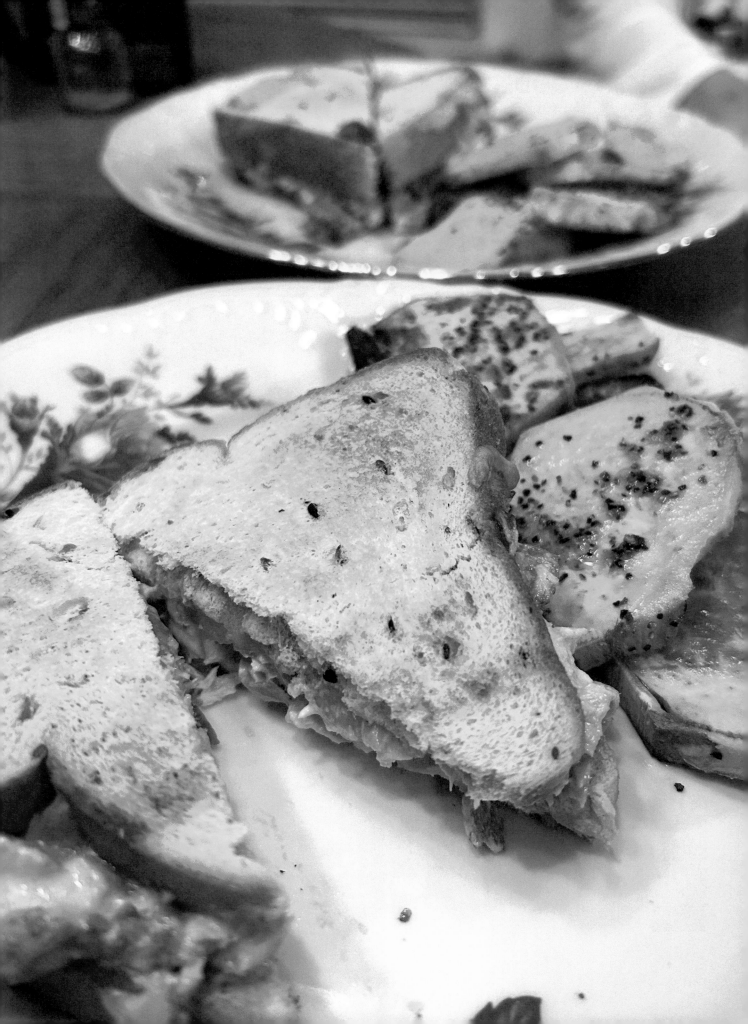

QUICK TUNA MELT OVEN

Serving Size:	2 servings	Cook time:	15 minutes
Prep time:	15 minutes	Needed:	Medium mixing bowl, baking sheet, spoon, spatula

DIRECTIONS

○ Preheat oven to 400° F.

dash ➤ Pepper, red, crushed
½ T ➤ Lemon Juice
2 ½ T ➤ Mayonnaise

○ In a medium mixing bowl, add the above ingredients and whisk together.

dash ➤ Black Pepper, ground
½ stalk ➤ Celery, fresh, chopped
1 T ➤ Parsley, fresh, chopped
dash ➤ Kosher Salt
2 T ➤ Onion, sweet, fresh, chopped
1 T ➤ Pickles, Dill, chopped
1 can ➤ Tuna, 5 oz can, drained

○ In same bowl, add the above ingredients.
Stir mixture until tuna is fully covered. Set aside.

4 slices ➤ Bread
1 T ➤ Butter
2 ➤ Cheese, Cheddar, slices
2 ➤ Tomato, medium, fresh, slices

○ Butter one side of each bread slice. Then place on baking sheet.
Top unbuttered side with half of the tuna mixture, tomato slice
and a slice of cheese. Top with another slice of bread (buttered side
facing up). Repeat with remaining ingredients and place on a large
baking sheet. Bake until cheese is melted (5–8 minutes). Serve warm.

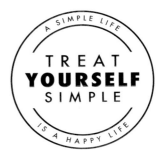

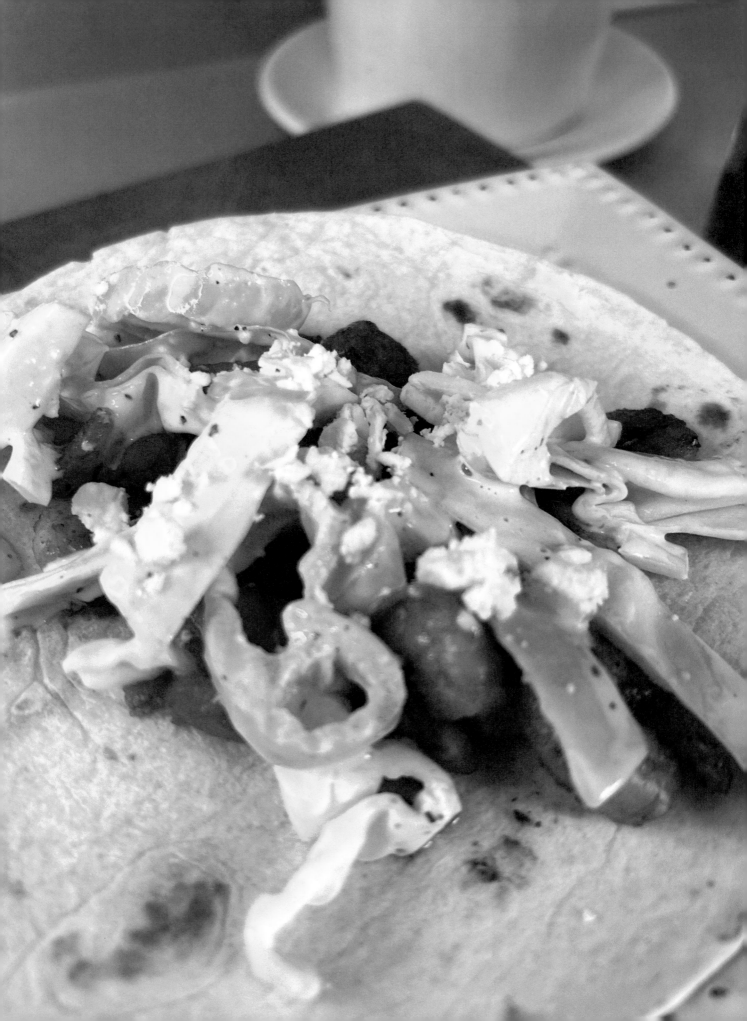

FETA SHRIMP TACOS STOVE

Serving Size:	2 servings	Cook time:	30 minutes
Prep time:	10 minutes	Needed:	Small mixing bowl, skillet, heat-safe spoon

DIRECTIONS

½ T ➤ Apple Cider Vinegar
dash ➤ Black Pepper, ground
2 T ➤ Mayonnaise
½ T ➤ Mustard

○ Combine above ingredients in mixing bowl.

½ ➤ Banana Pepper, chopped (if from a jar, ¼ C)
1 C ➤ Cabbage, red or green, fresh, shredded
2 T ➤ Onion, sweet, fresh, chopped

○ Add the above ingredients to same mixing bowl and toss to coat. Refrigerate slaw until serving.

½ T ➤ Olive Oil
12 ➤ Shrimp, large, peeled and deveined or 2 C Salad Shrimp
½ T ➤ Taco Seasoning

○ Coat skillet with olive oil over medium-low heat. Add shrimp and season with taco seasoning. Cook for 3–4 minutes until shrimp turns pink.

4 ➤ Tortilla Shells, 6–8", Flour or Corn
¼ C ➤ Cheese, Feta, crumbled
optional ➤ Avocado, fresh, sliced

○ Wrap tortillas in paper towels and heat in microwave for 30 seconds; Remove, unwrap, placing 2 tortillas on each of two plates. Divide shrimp evenly, top with the slaw, cheese and avocado. Serve warm.

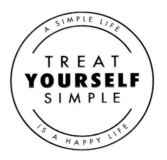

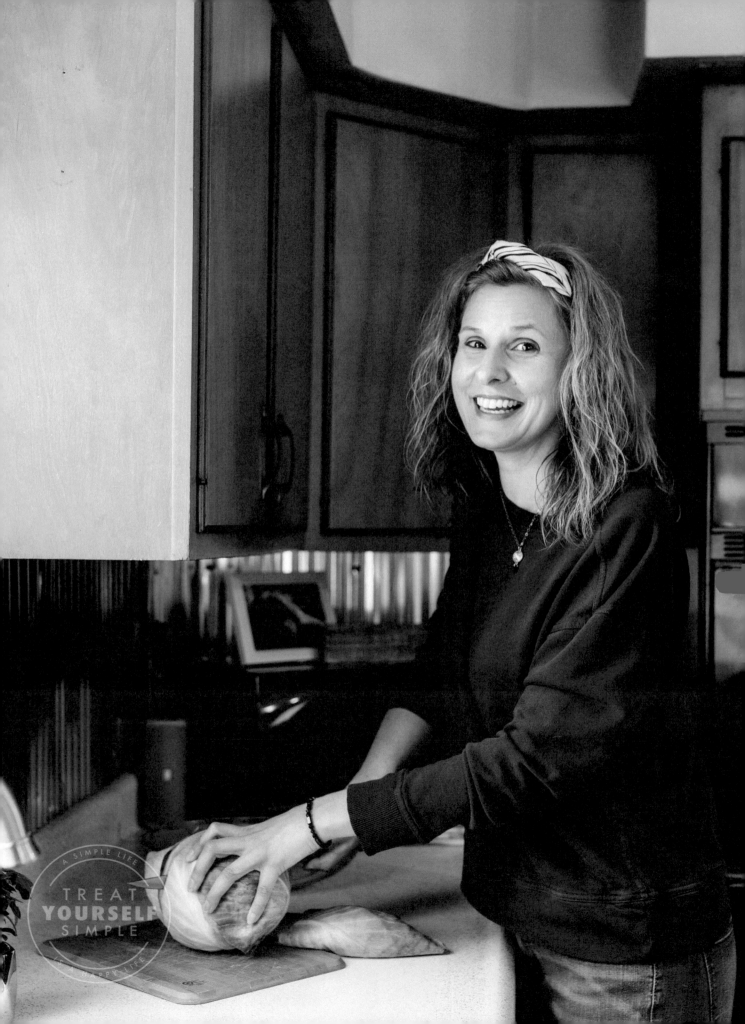

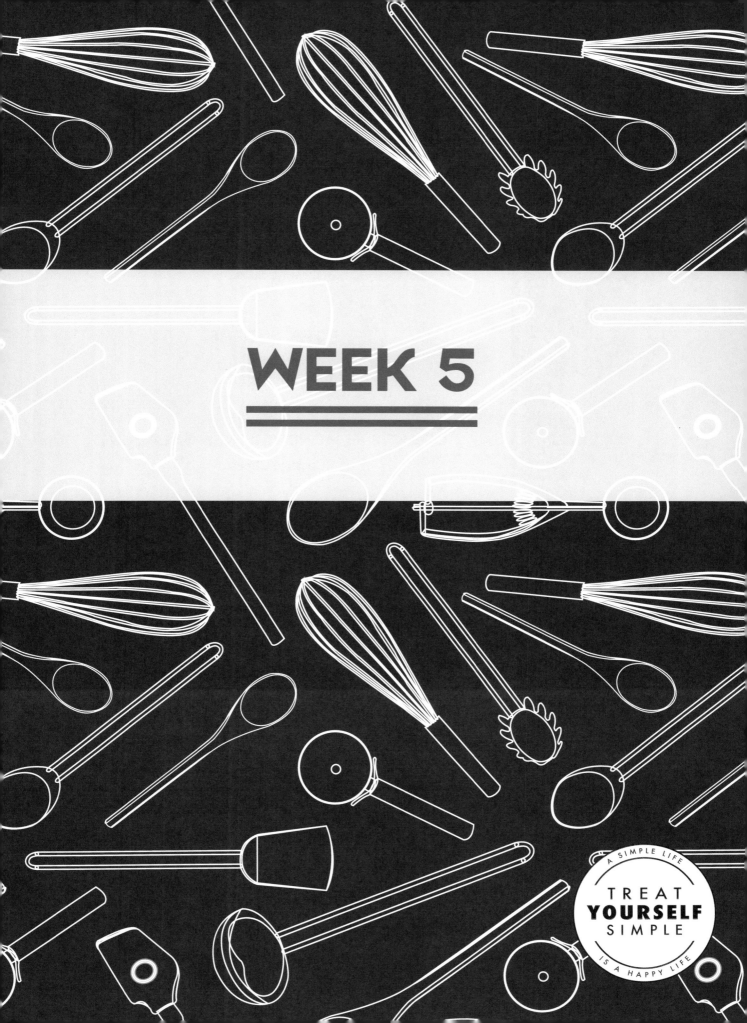

WEEK 5

TREAT
YOURSELF
SIMPLE

A SIMPLE LIFE

IS A HAPPY LIFE

WEEK 5 MENU PLAN

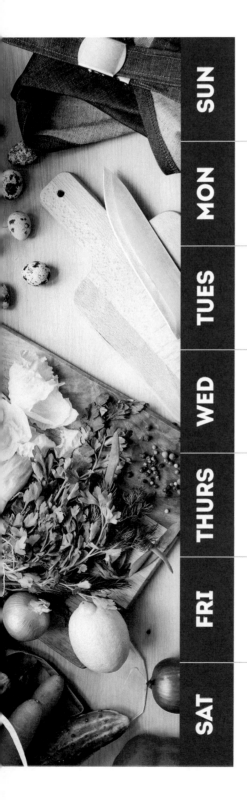

SUN

BUTTERNUT SQUASH SALAD

Sweet Potato Discs
Orange Slices

MON

PORK SLIDERS

Broccoli
Cinnamon Apples

TUES

ORANGE ALMOND CHICKEN SALAD 2/1

Cottage Cheese
Pears

WED

PESTO CHICKEN PITA

Corn
Fresh Fruit Bowl

THURS

BUDDHA BOWLS 2/1

Cucumber Slices
Cinnamon Apples

FRI

VEGETABLE BEEF SOUP

Fresh Salad
Orange Slices

SAT

SALMON BURGERS

Sweet Potato Discs
Pears

WEEK 5 GROCERY LIST

BUTTERNUT SQUASH SALAD

2 oz	Spinach, baby, fresh
dash	Black Pepper, ground
1¼ C	Squash, Butternut, cut into bite-sized pieces
2 T	Cheese, Feta, crumbled
¼ t	Thyme, fresh, chopped
2 T	Honey
dash	Kosher Salt
1 t	Mustard, Dijon
3 T	Olive Oil
1 T	Onions, green, fresh, sliced
¼ C	Walnuts, toasted, chopped
¼ C	Cranberries, dried
1 T	Red Wine Vinegar

PORK SLIDERS

¼	Avocado, fresh
4	Buns, Slider, lightly toasted
½ C	Cheese, Mozzarella, shredded
¼ t	Garlic, minced
2 t	Parsley, fresh
¼ t	Kosher Salt
1 t	Lemon Juice
4	Lettuce, Romaine leaves
½ lb	Pork, ground
1	Tomato, medium, fresh, sliced

ORANGE ALMOND CHICKEN SALAD 2/1

2 C	Spinach, baby, fresh
dash	Black Pepper, ground
4	Chicken Breasts, 4 oz each, 2 breasts for **Buddha Bowls 2/1**
dash	Kosher Salt
3 T	Almonds, sliced, toasted
2	Onions, green, fresh, sliced
1	Orange, fresh, peeled, sections, each slice halved
1 T	Olive Oil
2 T	Miso Ginger Dressing

PESTO CHICKEN PITA

2	Chicken Breasts, 4 oz each, cut into bite-sized pieces
¼	Onion, red, fresh, cut into 1" pieces
1	Bell Pepper, any color, fresh, cut into 1" pieces
1	Zucchini, fresh, cut into 1" pieces
1 T	Olive Oil
dash	Kosher Salt
dash	Black Pepper, ground
2½ T	Pesto, store-bought
1	Pita, halved

BUDDHA BOWLS 2/1

½ C	Avocado, fresh, sliced
1 C	Spinach, baby, fresh
dash	Black Pepper, ground
2	Chicken Breasts, 4 oz each, from **Orange Almond Chicken Salad 2/1**
½ T	Cilantro, fresh, chopped
¼ t	Garlic, minced
¼"	Ginger, fresh, peeled, grated
dash	Kosher Salt
2 t	Olive Oil
½ C	Onion, red, fresh, chopped
1 C	Rice, Jasmine
½ t	Sesame Seeds, toasted, white
1	Sweet Potato, large, peeled, cut into bite-sized pieces
	Miso Ginger Dressing, purchased at store

BY MEAL

VEGETABLE BEEF SOUP

½ C	Vegetables, mixed, frozen
1 ½ T	Olive Oil
½ lb	Beef Stew meat, cubed
¼ t	Kosher Salt
¼ t	Black Pepper, ground
¼ C	Onion, sweet, chopped
1 t	Garlic, minced
1 stalk	Celery, large/long, chopped
3	Carrots, chopped
2 T	Flour
2 ¾ C	Broth, Vegetable
1 ⅛ C	Water
1 T	Tomato Paste
1	Bay leaf
1 T	Thyme, fresh or 1 t dried
1	Potato, diced
½ C	Mushrooms, cooked, optional

SALMON BURGERS

dash	Black Pepper, ground
2	Buns, Brioche, lightly toasted
dash	Cayenne Pepper
dash	Kosher Salt
¼ t	Lemon Juice
½ T	Mayonnaise
1 T	Mustard, Dijon
1	Onion, green, chopped
optional	Lettuce, Romaine, fresh
2	Salmon Patties, 4 oz, frozen, pre-made
optional	Tartar Sauce

WEEK 5 PREP

Mince 5 Garlic Cloves ~ Pork Sliders; Buddha Bowls 2/1, Vegetable Beef Soup

Cut 2 Chicken Breasts into bite-sized pieces ~ Pesto Chicken Pita

Chop 1 Bell Pepper, any color, fresh ~ Pesto Chicken Pita

Buy or Cut 1 ¼ C Butternut Squash into bite-sized pieces ~ Butternut Squash Salad

Chop 3 Carrots ~ Vegetable Beef Soup

Chop 1 Celery stalk ~ Vegetable Beef Soup

Chop ¾ Onion, red, fresh ~ Pesto Chicken Pita; Buddha Bowls 2/1

Chop ¼ Onion, sweet ~ Vegetable Beef Soup

Cut 1 large Sweet Potato into bite-sized pieces ~ Buddha Bowls 2/1

Chop 1 ½ Zucchini, fresh ~ Pesto Chicken Pita, Butternut Squash Salad

Shred ½ C Mozzarella Cheese ~ Pork Sliders

WEEK 5 MAKE AHEAD

Make 1 C Jasmine Rice ~ Buddha Bowls 2/1

Bake 1 ¼ C Butternut Squash ~ Butternut Squash Salad

Buy or Chop ¼ C Walnuts, then toast ~ Butternut Squash Salad

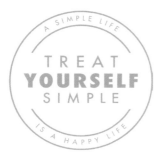

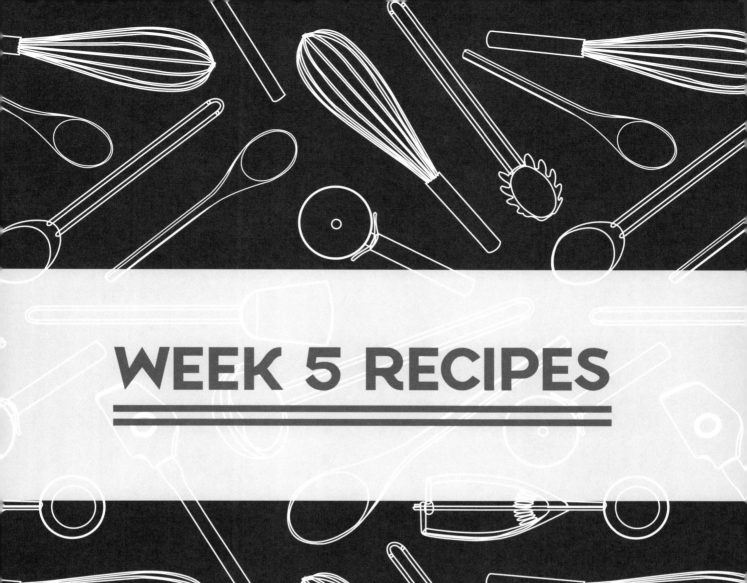

WEEK 5 RECIPES

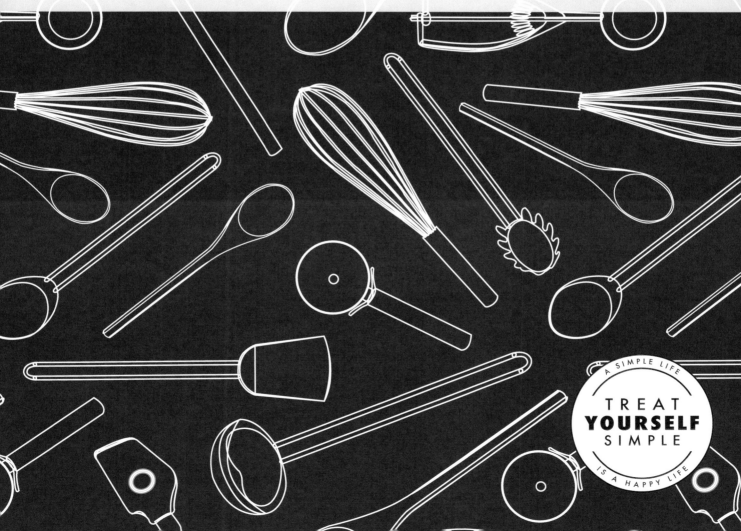

A SIMPLE LIFE

TREAT
YOURSELF
SIMPLE

IS A HAPPY LIFE

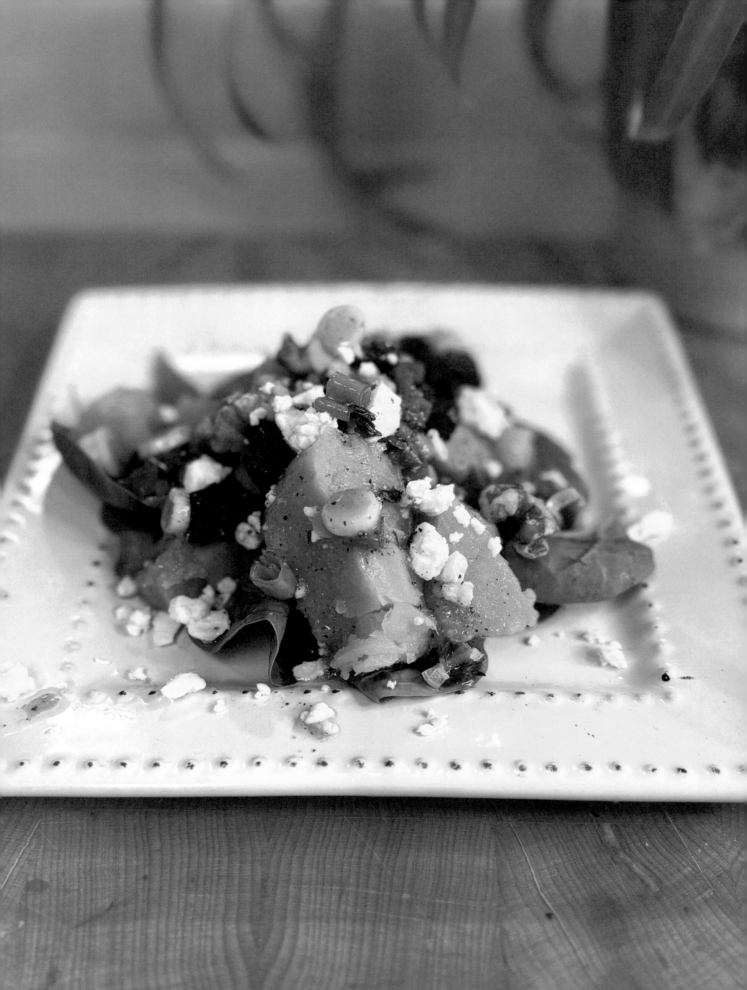

BUTTERNUT SQUASH SALAD OVEN + NO COOK

Serving Size:	2 servings	Cook time:	25 minutes
Prep time:	20 minutes	Needed:	Medium mixing bowl, measuring cup or small bowl, baking sheet, spatula

DIRECTIONS

1¼ C ➤ Squash, Butternut, cut into bite-sized pieces
1 T ➤ Olive Oil
dash ➤ Kosher Salt
dash ➤ Black Pepper, ground

○ If squash is not cooked, preheat oven to 400° F.

○ Spread pieces across foil lined baking sheet, drizzle with olive oil and season with salt & pepper. Toss evenly to coat; then spread into an even layer. Bake for 15 minutes; remove from oven and toss. Return to oven and bake until tender, about 10 minutes longer. Allow to cool before adding to the salad. Can be made ahead.

2 T ➤ Olive Oil
1 T ➤ Red Wine Vinegar
1 T ➤ Onions, green, fresh, sliced
2 T ➤ Honey
1 t ➤ Mustard, Dijon
¼ t ➤ Thyme, fresh, chopped
dash ➤ Kosher Salt
dash ➤ Black Pepper, ground

○ Combine above ingredients in a measuring cup or small bowl; whisk until combined. Set aside.

¼ C ➤ Walnuts, toasted, chopped
2 oz ➤ Spinach, baby, fresh
¼ C ➤ Cranberries, dried
2 T ➤ Cheese, Feta, crumbled

○ Combine half of the pecans, half of the cranberries, and squash in medium mixing bowl. Divide spinach between two plates. Divide squash mixture on spinach on each plate. Drizzle with dressing. Sprinkle with remaining half of the pecans, half of the cranberries, and cheese. Serve cold immediately.

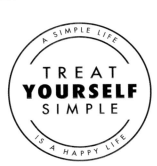

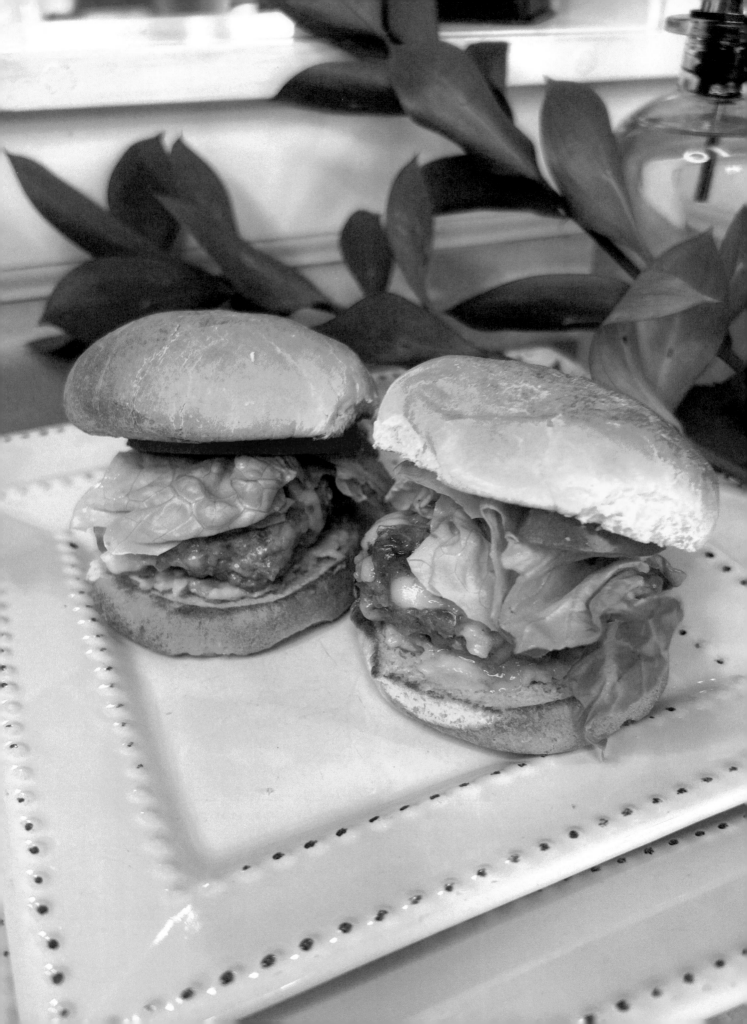

PORK SLIDERS STOVE

Serving Size:	2 servings	Cook time:	15 minutes
Prep time:	10 minutes	Needed:	Large skillet, medium mixing bowl, small mixing bowl, heat-safe spoon

DIRECTIONS

¼ t ➤ Garlic, minced
2 t ➤ Parsley, fresh, chopped
¼ t ➤ Kosher Salt
½ lb ➤ Pork, ground

○ Combine the above ingredients in a medium mixing bowl; mix with hands; divide into four equal parts, shaping into ¼ inch thick patties.
Coat a large skillet, with cooking spray.

○ Over medium-high heat, add patties and cook for 5–10 minutes.
Cook patties flipping once, until internal temperature reaches 160° F.

½ C ➤ Cheese, Mozzarella, shredded

○ Add shredded cheese to patties and cook until melted. Turn off heat.

¼ ➤ Avocado, fresh
1 t ➤ Lemon Juice

○ Combine the above ingredients in a small mixing bowl.
Mash with a fork and mix thoroughly. Set aside.

4 ➤ Buns, Slider, lightly toasted
4 ➤ Lettuce, Romaine, small leaves
1 ➤ Tomato, medium, fresh, sliced

○ Place two buns on each of two plates. Divide, over bottom half of each bun, the spread, a patty, a lettuce leaf, and tomato slice; place top half of bun to make slider. Serve warm.

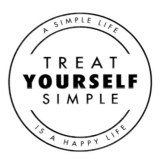

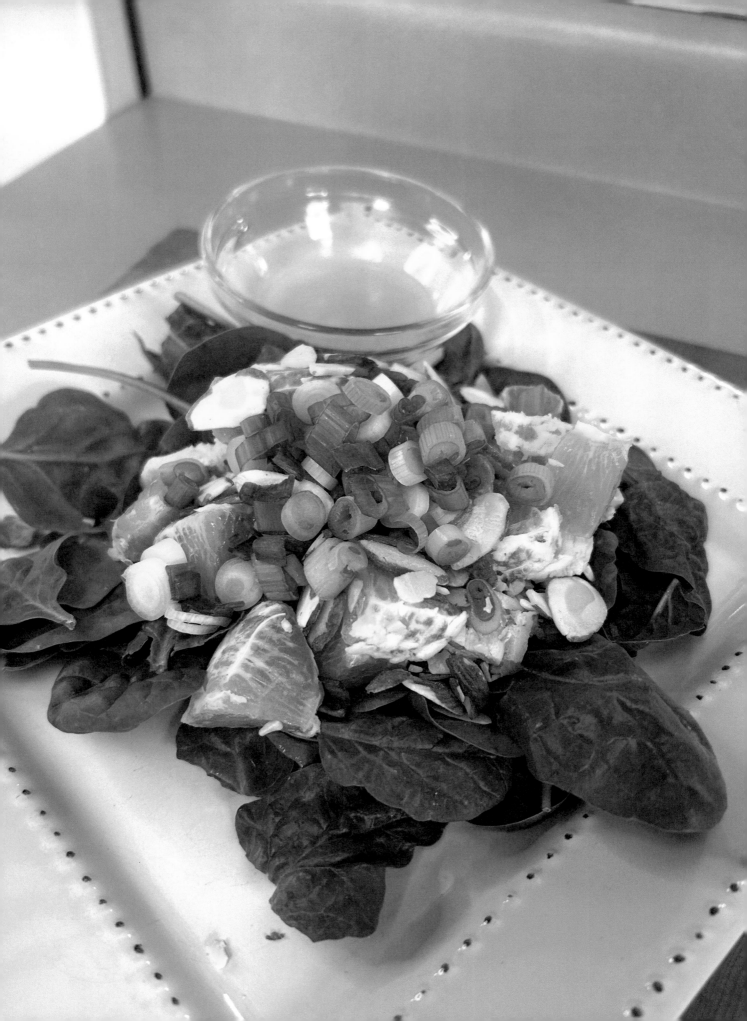

ORANGE ALMOND CHICKEN SALAD 2/1 STOVE

Please note: Makes Chicken for Buddha Bowls 2/1

Serving Size:	2 servings	Cook time:	12 minutes
Prep time:	12 minutes	Needed:	Large skillet, olive oil, spatula

DIRECTIONS

1 T ➤ Olive Oil
4 ➤ Chicken Breasts, 4 oz each
dash ➤ Black Pepper, ground
dash ➤ Kosher Salt

○ Coat skillet with olive oil over medium-high heat. Add chicken, season with salt & pepper; cook for 8–12 minutes, flipping at least once until internal temperature reaches 165° F. Remove from heat. Cut 2 chicken breasts into bite-sized pieces.

NOTE: *Remove two of the chicken breasts for* **Buddha Bowls 2/1.** *Set aside, cool, and store in an airtight container. Refrigerate for 7–10 days.*

2 C ➤ Spinach, baby, fresh
3 T ➤ Almonds, sliced, toasted
2 ➤ Onions, green, fresh, sliced
1 ➤ Orange, fresh, peeled, sections, each slice halved
2 T ➤ Miso Ginger Dressing

○ Place spinach into each of two bowls, add chicken; top with almonds, onion, and orange. Drizzle dressing over salad. Serve immediately.

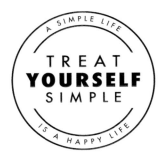

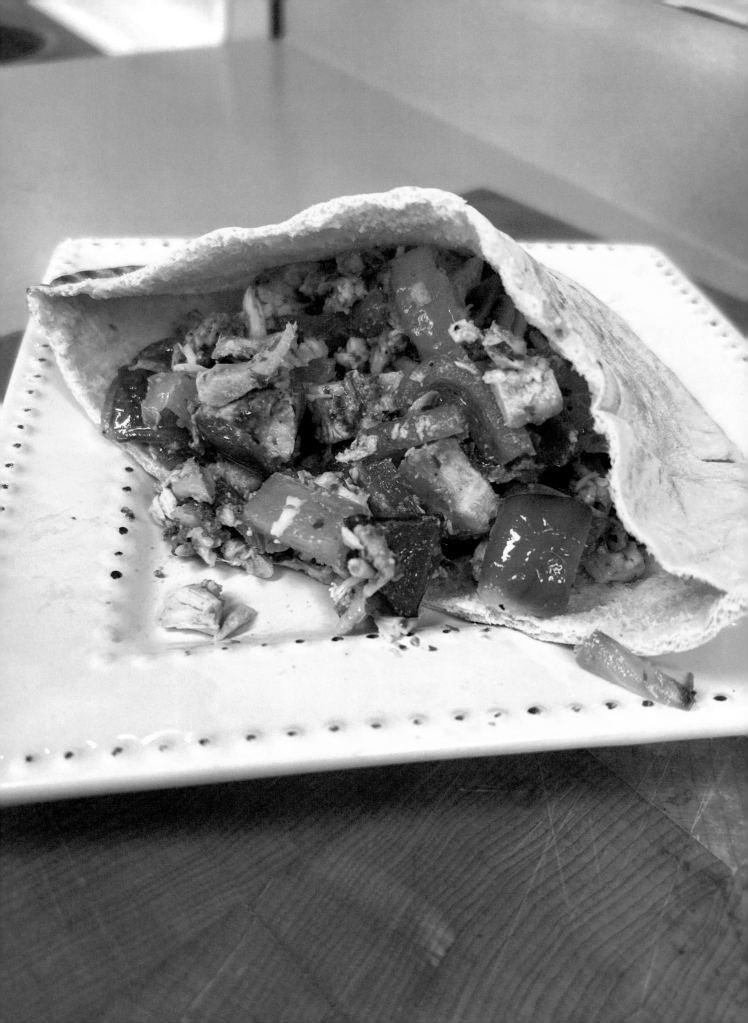

PESTO CHICKEN PITA OVEN

Serving Size:	2 servings	Cook time:	15 minutes
Prep time:	10 minutes	Needed:	Baking sheet, large bowl, spatula

DIRECTIONS

○ Heat oven to 425° F. Coat foil-lined baking sheet with cooking spray.

2 ➤ Chicken Breasts, 4 oz each, cut into bite-sized pieces
¼ ➤ Onion, red, fresh, cut into 1" pieces
1 ➤ Bell Pepper, any color, fresh, cut into 1" pieces
1 ➤ Zucchini, fresh, cut into 1" pieces
1 T ➤ Olive Oil
dash ➤ Kosher Salt
dash ➤ Black Pepper, ground

○ Toss the chicken and vegetable with olive oil and salt & pepper in a large bowl; arrange on prepared baking sheet; cook for 10 minutes; flip chicken and vegetables and return to the oven; cook 10 minutes. Return to bowl.

2 ½ T ➤ Pesto, store-bought

○ Add pesto to chicken and vegetable mixture, stir to coat.

1 ➤ Bread, Pita, halved

○ Divide between pita halves. Serve warm or cold.

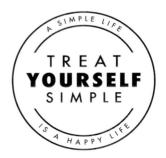

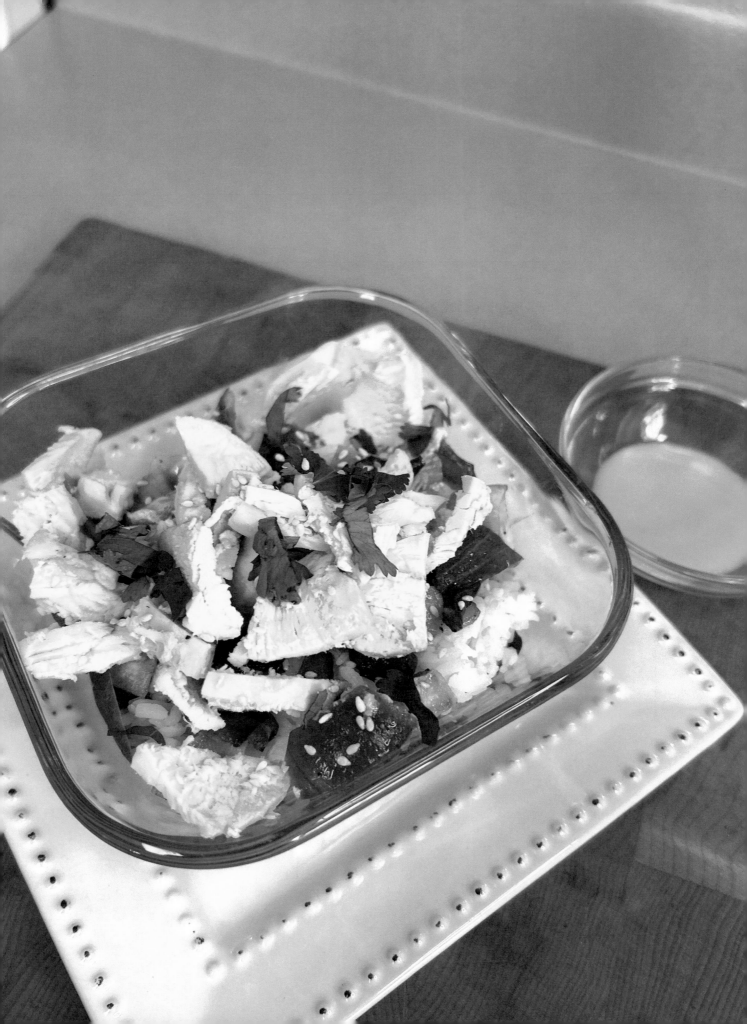

BUDDHA BOWLS 2/1 OVEN

Please note: Chicken was prepared from Orange Almond Chicken Salad 2/1

Serving Size:	2 servings	**Cook time:**	30 minutes
Prep time:	10 minutes	**Needed:**	Baking sheet, medium saucepan, large skillet, heat-safe spoon

DIRECTIONS

○ Preheat over to 425° F. Coat a baking sheet with olive oil.

dash ➤ Black Pepper, ground
dash ➤ Kosher Salt
1 t ➤ Olive Oil
½ C ➤ Onion, red, fresh, chopped
1 ➤ Sweet Potato, large, peeled, cut into bite-sized pieces

○ **Sweet Potato Mixture:** Toss above ingredients onto baking sheet.
Bake until tender (20–25 minutes).

1 C ➤ Rice, Jasmine

○ **Can make ahead. See Make Ahead Directions.** If not already prepared, prepare rice according to package instructions. Set aside.

2 ➤ Chicken Breasts, 4 oz each, from **Orange Almond Chicken Salad 2/1**
¼ t ➤ Garlic, minced
¼" ➤ Ginger, fresh, peeled and grated
1 t ➤ Olive Oil

○ While rice is cooking, coat skillet with olive oil over medium-high heat.
Cut chicken breasts into bite-sized pieces. Add above ingredients to skillet.
Cook until heated through, about 5–7 minutes.

½ C ➤ Avocado, fresh, sliced
1 C ➤ Spinach, baby, fresh
½ T ➤ Cilantro, fresh, chopped
½ t ➤ Sesame Seeds, toasted, white
➤ Miso Ginger Dressing, purchased at store

○ Divide rice among two bowls and top each with sweet potato mixture, remaining chicken, avocado, and baby spinach.
Sprinkle with cilantro and sesame seeds.
Drizzle with dressing before serving. Serve immediately.

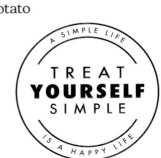

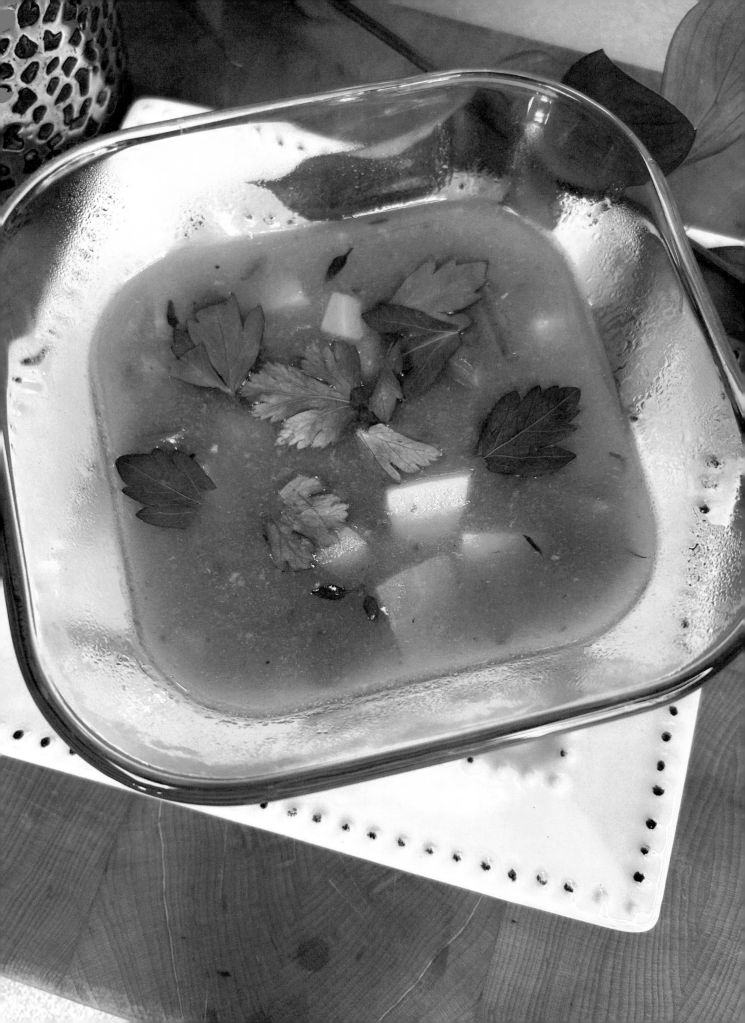

VEGETABLE BEEF SOUP STOVE

Serving Size:	2 servings	Cook time:	1–1 ½ hours
Prep time:	10 minutes	Needed:	Medium saucepan, mixing bowl, heat-safe spoon

DIRECTIONS

1 T ➤ Olive Oil

○ Add oil to pan over medium-high heat.

½ lb ➤ Beef stew meat, cubed
¼ t ➤ Kosher Salt
¼ t ➤ Black Pepper, ground

○ Add beef to medium saucepan. Season with salt & pepper. Brown beef for 3–5 minutes. Remove from pan and place in mixing bowl. Set aside.

½ T ➤ Olive Oil
¼ C ➤ Onion, sweet, chopped
1 t ➤ Garlic, minced
1 stalk ➤ Celery, large/long, chopped
3 ➤ Carrots, chopped

○ Turn heat to medium. Add above ingredients to pan, cooking for 4 minutes, until onion is translucent.

2 T ➤ Flour
2 ¾ C ➤ Broth, Vegetable
1 ⅛ C ➤ Water
1 T ➤ Tomato Paste
1 ➤ Bay leaf
1 T ➤ Thyme, fresh or 1 t dried
1 ➤ Potato, diced

○ Stir in flour, then slowly pour in beef broth while constantly stirring. Add the rest of the above ingredients. Add the browned beef. Stir to combine. Cook until gently boiling. Turn down heat to simmer, cover, cook for 1 hour 15 minutes.

½ C ➤ Vegetables, mixed, frozen
½ C ➤ Mushrooms, cooked, optional

○ Add the mixed vegetables. Bring to boil. Simmer for 5 minutes, uncovered.

➤ Parsley, to garnish

○ Ladle into bowls. Sprinkle with parsley. Serve warm.

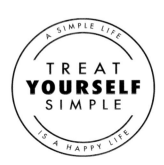

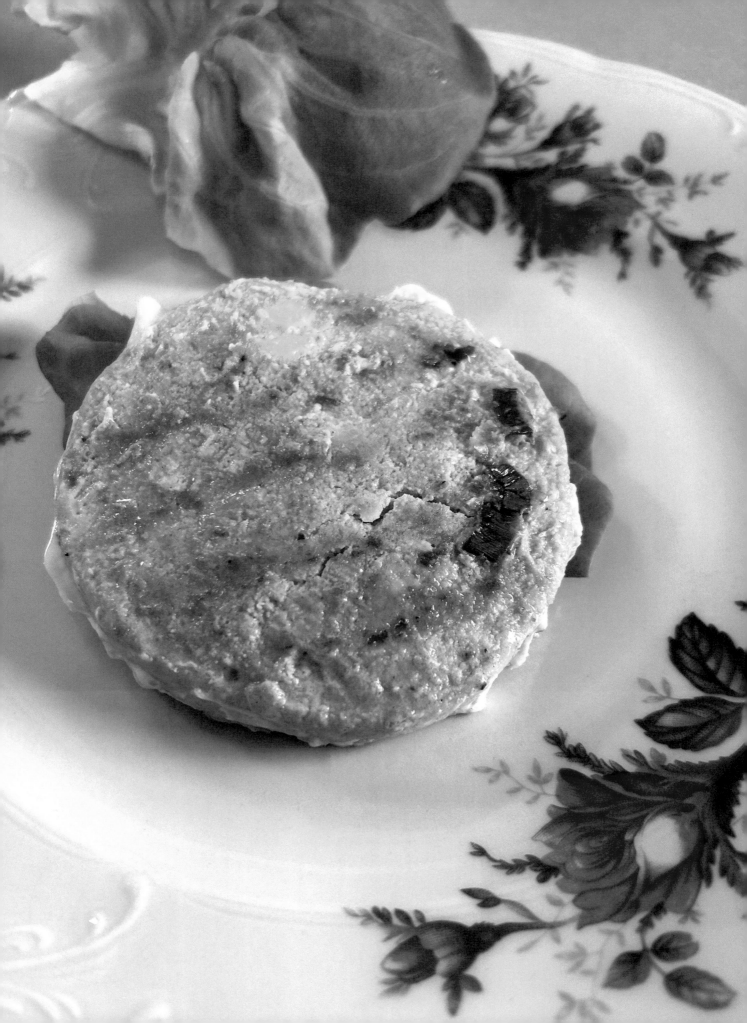

SALMON BURGERS OVEN

Serving Size:	2 servings	Cook time:	20 minutes
Prep time:	10 minutes	Needed:	Medium mixing bowls, baking sheet, spatula

DIRECTIONS

○ Preheat oven to 400° F. Line baking sheet with aluminum foil and coat with cooking spray. Set aside.

dash ➤ Black Pepper, ground
dash ➤ Cayenne Pepper
dash ➤ Kosher Salt
¼ t ➤ Lemon Juice
½ T ➤ Mayonnaise
1 T ➤ Mustard, Dijon
1 ➤ Onion, green, chopped
2 ➤ Salmon Patties, 4 oz, frozen, premade

○ Combine the above ingredients in a medium mixing bowl.
Coat both sides of each patty with mix. Place on lined baking sheet.
Bake for 20 minutes until internal temperature reaches 145° F.
Remove from heat.

2 ➤ Buns, Brioche, lightly toasted
optional ➤ Lettuce, Romaine, fresh
optional ➤ Tartar Sauce

○ On each of two plates, place bottom bun, top with prepared salmon patty, optional ingredients, and top of bun. Serve warm.

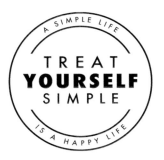

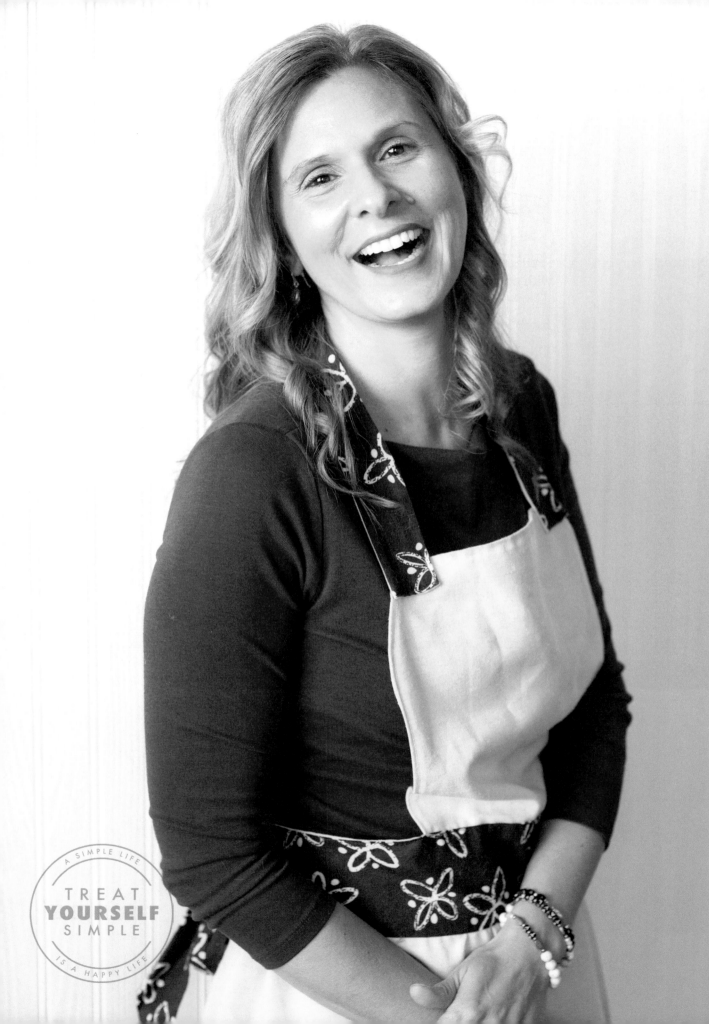

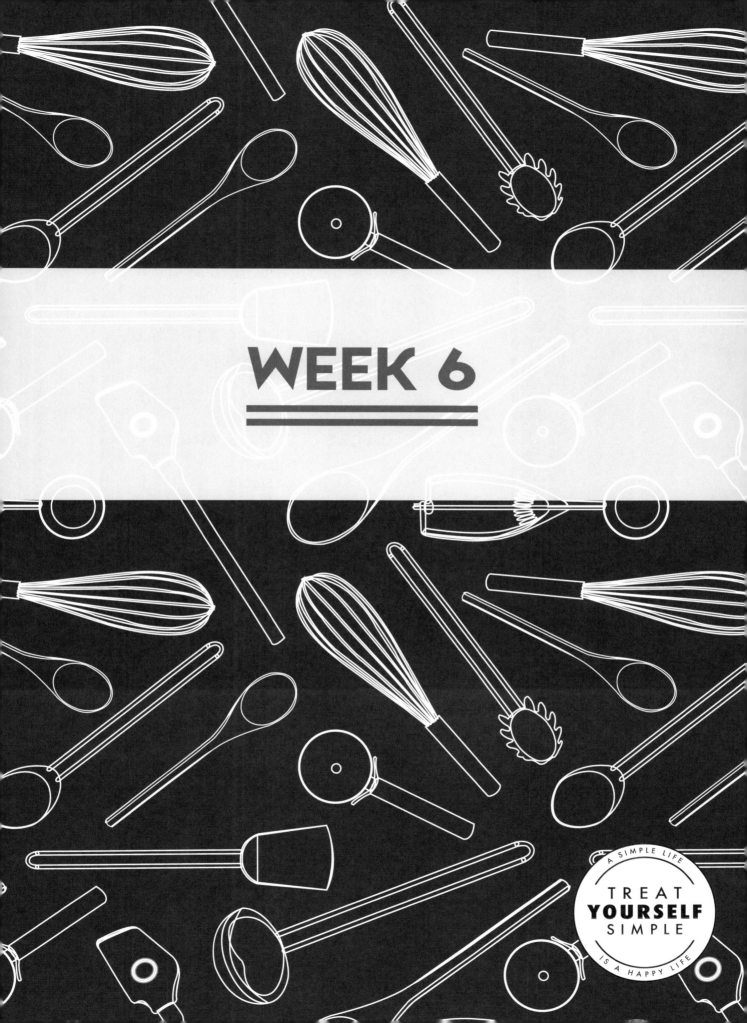

WEEK 6

WEEK 6 MENU PLAN

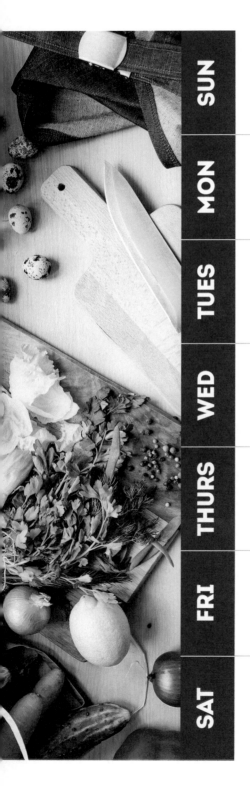

SUN

FALL HARVEST SALAD

Crackers
Apple Slices

MON

FULLY LOADED BREAKFAST TACOS

Guacamole and Chips
Pears

TUES

CHICKEN LETTUCE WRAPS

Quinoa
Brussel Sprouts

WED

CILANTRO LIME SHRIMP

Sweet Potato Discs
Coleslaw

THURS

BROCCOLI CHEDDAR CHICKEN CASSEROLE 2/1

Coleslaw
Cinnamon Apples

FRI

CHICKEN ENCHILADA STUFFED SQUASH

Fresh Salad
Pears

SAT

CHICKEN SPINACH SALAD 2/1

Cornbread
Pears

WEEK 6 GROCERY LIST

FALL HARVEST SALAD

2 t	Apple Cider Vinegar
1	Apple, Honey Crisp, fresh, diced
2 C	Spinach, baby, fresh
dash	Black Pepper, ground
dash	Cinnamon, ground
1 oz	Deli Ham, thinly sliced
2 T	Cheese, Feta
1 t	Thyme, fresh, chopped
dash	Kosher Salt
1 t	Maple Syrup
2 t	Olive Oil
1	Onion, green, sliced
1½ T	Pumpkin Seeds
optional	Pepper, red, crushed

FULLY LOADED BREAKFAST TACOS

optional	Avocado, fresh, chopped
2 slices	Bacon, crumbled or 2 T Real Bacon Bits/Crumbles
dash	Black Pepper, ground
optional	Cheese, Mexican, shredded
dash	Pepper, red, crushed
¼ t	Cumin, ground
3	Eggs
dash	Garlic Powder
1 t	Cilantro, fresh
dash	Kosher Salt
1 t	Lime Juice
1 t	Olive Oil
1 T	Onion, red, chopped
1	Potatoes, Russet, large, diced
dash	Seasoning Salt
1 T	Sour Cream
1/3 C	Tomatoes, medium, fresh, chopped
4	Tortilla Shells, 6-8", Flour or Carn, warmed
	Salsa
optional	Cilantro, fresh, chopped

CHICKEN LETTUCE WRAPS

1 T + 1 t	Garlic, minced
½ T + ½ T	Ginger, fresh, peeled, minced or ¼ t ground Ginger
1 T + 1½ T	Soy Sauce
1 T	Rice Vinegar
¾ T + ½ T	Sesame Oil
½ T	Honey
3 T	Olive Oil
½ lb	Chicken, ground
2 T	Hoisin Sauce
1 T	Rice Vinegar
½ T	Pepper, red, crushed
1	Onion, green, chopped
¼ C	Water Chestnuts, diced
	Lettuce, butter or Romaine, wide leaf
½ C	Carrots, shredded
½ C	Cucumber halves, sliced
½ C	Almonds, slivered
½	Avocado, large, diced

CILANTRO LIME SHRIMP

dash	Black Pepper, ground
1 T	Cilantro, fresh, chopped
2 C	Corn, frozen
½ t	Pepper, red, crushed
1 t	Cumin, ground
1½ t	Garlic, minced
dash	Kosher Salt
½ t	Olive Oil
12	Shrimp, large, peeled and deveined or 2 C Salad Shrimp
1 T	Butter
1	Lime, sliced into rounds

BY MEAL

BROCCOLI CHEDDAR CHICKEN CASSEROLE 2/1

1	Bay leaf
dash	Black Pepper, ground
1 T	Butter
½ C	Carrot, shredded
¼ t	Cayenne Pepper
¾ C	Cheese, Cheddar, sharp, shredded
4	Chicken Breasts, 4 oz each, cut into bite-sized pieces, 2 breasts for **Chicken Enchilada Stuffed Squash 2/1**
1½ C	Broth, Chicken
¼ t	Garlic Powder
1 T	Thyme, fresh, chopped
dash	Kosher Salt
1 T	Lemon Juice
¼ C	Milk
½ T	Olive Oil
½ C	Onion, sweet, chopped
2 oz	Pasta, orzo
1 C	Rice, Jasmine
1½ C	Broccoli florets, frozen

CHICKEN ENCHILADA STUFFED SQUASH 2/1

1	Squash, Acorn, small, halved, seeds removed
½ T	Olive Oil
2 T	Onion, sweet, fresh, chopped
1 t	Garlic, minced
¼ t	Cumin, ground
dash	Kosher Salt
dash	Black Pepper, ground
½ can	Enchilada Sauce, red, 10 oz can
2	Chicken Breasts, 4 oz each, cut into bite-sized pieces, from **Broccoli Cheddar Chicken Casserole 2/1**
¼ C	Cilantro, fresh, chopped
½ C	Cheese, Cheddar, shredded
optional	Sour Cream

CHICKEN SPINACH SALAD

½ t	Mustard, Dijon
½ t	Honey
1 t	Red Wine Vinegar
2 T	Olive Oil
dash	Kosher Salt
dash	Black Pepper, ground
1	Apple, cubed
⅓ C	Cheese, Cheddar, shredded
2	Chicken Breasts, 4 oz each
¼ C	Pumpkin Seeds
2 C	Spinach

WEEK 6 PREP

Mince 13 Garlic Cloves ~ Chicken Lettuce Wraps, Cilantro Lime Shrimp, Chicken Enchilada Stuffed Squash

Cut Chicken Breast into bite-sized pieces ~ Broccoli Cheddar Chicken Casserole 2/1, Chicken Spinach Salad 2/1

Chop ⅛ Red Onion ~ Fully Loaded Breakfast Tacos

Chop ½ Sweet Onion ~ Chicken Enchilada Stuffed Squash, Broccoli Cheddar Chicken Casserole 2/1

Shred 1½ C Sharp Cheddar Cheese ~ Broccoli Cheddar Chicken Casserole 2/1, Chicken Spinach Salad 2/1, Chicken Enchilada Stuffed Squash

Chop ½ Tomato ~ Fully Loaded Breakfast Tacos

Chop 2 Green Onions ~ Fall Harvest Salad, Chicken Lettuce Wraps

Shred 2 Carrots ~ Chicken Lettuce Wraps, Broccoli Cheddar Chicken Casserole 2/1

WEEK 6 MAKE AHEAD

Bake 1 Acorn Squash ~ Chicken Enchilada Stuffed Squash

Cook 2 slices of Bacon ~ Fully Loaded Breakfast Tacos

Make Dressing ~ Fall Harvest Salad, Chicken Lettuce Wraps, Chicken Spinach Salad 2/1

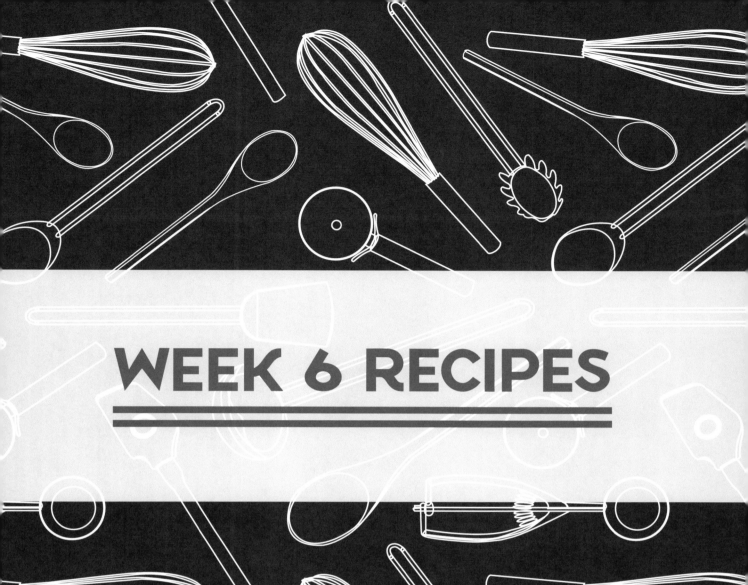
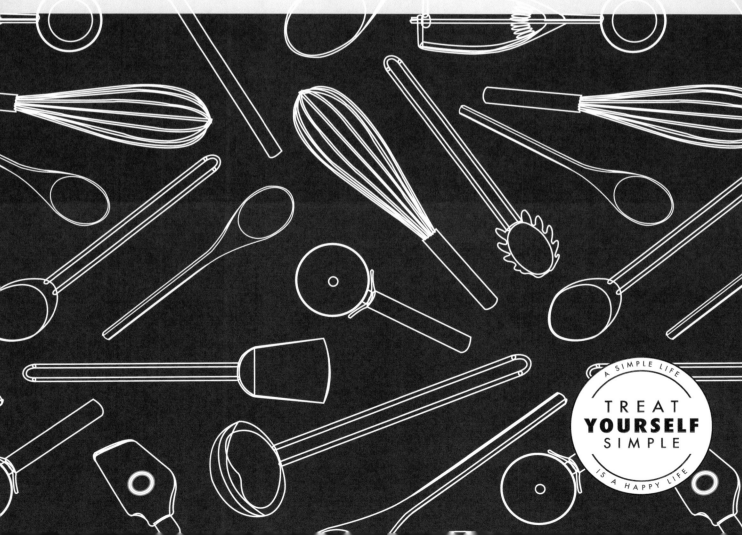

WEEK 6 RECIPES

A SIMPLE LIFE
TREAT
YOURSELF
SIMPLE
IS A HAPPY LIFE

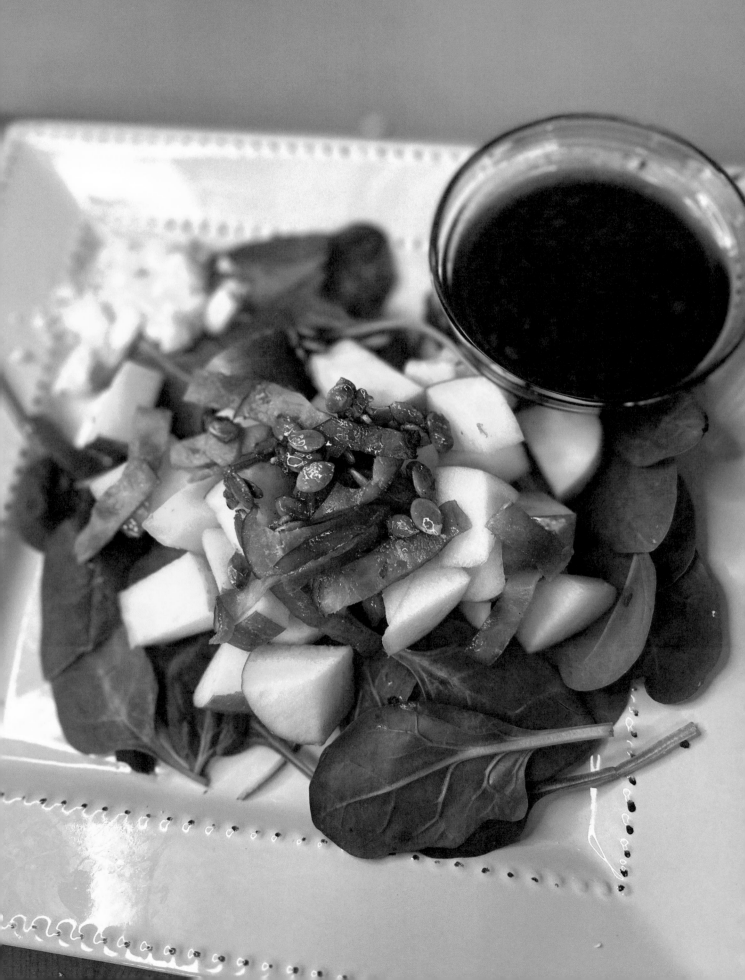

FALL HARVEST SALAD OVEN

Serving Size:	2 servings	Cook time:	15 minutes
Prep time:	15 minutes	Needed:	Baking sheet, foil, cooking spray, spatula, small bowl or measuring cup, large, mixing bowl, whisk, spatula

DIRECTIONS

○ Preheat oven to 350° F.

○ Line baking sheet with aluminum foil. Coat with coating spray.

2 t ➤ Apple Cider Vinegar
1 t ➤ Olive Oil
dash ➤ Black Pepper, ground
optional ➤ Pepper, red, crushed
1 t ➤ Thyme, fresh, chopped
dash ➤ Kosher Salt

DRESSING

○ **Can make ahead. See Make Ahead Directions.** If not already prepared, Add the above ingredients in a small bowl or measuring cup; whisk together until well blended. Refrigerate until ready to serve.

dash ➤ Cinnamon, ground
dash ➤ Kosher Salt
1 t ➤ Maple Syrup
1 t ➤ Olive Oil
1 oz ➤ Deli Ham, thinly sliced
1½ T ➤ Pumpkin Seeds

○ In a small mixing bowl, toss together the pumpkin seeds, olive oil, maple syrup, cinnamon, and salt. Spread pumpkin seed mixture in a single layer on prepared baking sheet; lay the deli ham flat around pumpkin seed mixture. Bake for 10–15 minutes or until the pumpkin seeds are toasted and the deli ham is crisp.

1 ➤ Apple, Honey Crisp, fresh, diced
2 C ➤ Spinach, baby, fresh
1 ➤ Onion, green, sliced

○ In a large mixing bowl, toss the spinach and apple together, set aside.

2 T ➤ Cheese, Feta

○ Divide salad mixture in two bowls or on two plates; top each with half of the ham, pumpkin seed mixture and feta cheese. Drizzle dressing over contents of each bowl or plate. Serve immediately.

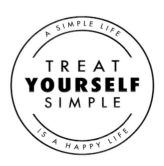

A SIMPLE LIFE
TREAT
YOURSELF
SIMPLE
IS A HAPPY LIFE

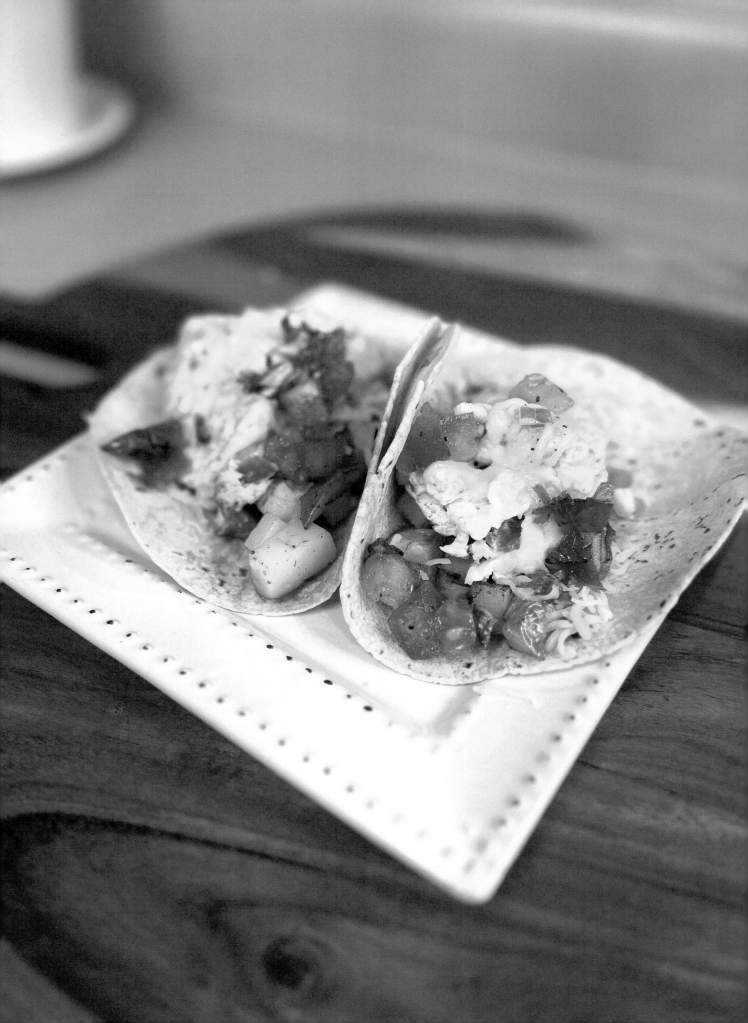

FULLY LOADED BREAKFAST TACOS STOVE

Serving Size:	2 servings	Cook time:	25–35 minutes
Prep time:	10 minutes	Needed:	Two small bowls, two forks, large skillet, baking sheet, plate, paper towel, spatula

DIRECTIONS

dash ➤ Black Pepper, ground
1 t ➤ Cilantro, fresh, chopped
dash ➤ Kosher Salt
1 t ➤ Lime Juice
1 t ➤ Olive Oil
1 t ➤ Onion, red, chopped
⅓ C ➤ Tomatoes, medium, fresh, chopped

○ Combine the above ingredients in small bowl, stirring together. Set aside.

dash ➤ Garlic Powder
1 ➤ Potato, Russet, large, diced
dash ➤ Seasoning Salt

○ Coat large skillet with olive oil over medium heat. Add the above ingredients; cook, stirring occasionally, until potatoes are crispy about 8–10 minutes. Turn heat off; remove from skillet; set aside.

2 slices ➤ Bacon, crumbled or 2 T Real Bacon Bits/Crumbles

○ **Can make ahead. See Make Ahead Directions.** If not already prepared, preheat oven to 375º F. Line baking sheet with aluminum foil. Place bacon slices on baking sheet. Bake for 25 minutes.

○ Remove from oven and baking sheet. Line paper towels to a plate. Place cooked bacon slices on paper towels to drain grease. Let cool for about 5 minutes. Crumble bacon or cut into small pieces with kitchen scissors. Set aside to use for garnish. Refrigerate any extra for 7–10 days and use for other meals.

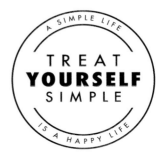

dash ➤ Pepper, red, crushed
¼ t ➤ Cumin, ground
3 ➤ Eggs
1 T ➤ Sour Cream

○ Add the above ingredients and bacon crumbles in a small bowl;
whisk together until blended. Coat same skillet with olive oil over medium heat.
Add egg mixture; cook for 5–8 minutes, stirring frequently, until eggs
are fully cooked.

4 ➤ Tortilla Shells, 6–8", Flour or Corn, warmed
➤ Salsa
optional ➤ Avocado, fresh, chopped
optional ➤ Cheese, Mexican, shredded
optional ➤ Cilantro, fresh, chopped

○ Wrap tortillas in paper towels and heat in microwave for 30 seconds;
Remove, unwrap, placing 2 tortillas each on two plates.
Divide potato mixture and egg mixture between evenly.
Top with, salsa, and optional ingredients. Serve warm.

NOTES

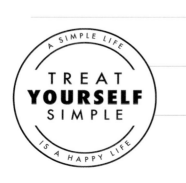

TREAT
YOURSELF
SIMPLE
A SIMPLE LIFE
IS A HAPPY LIFE

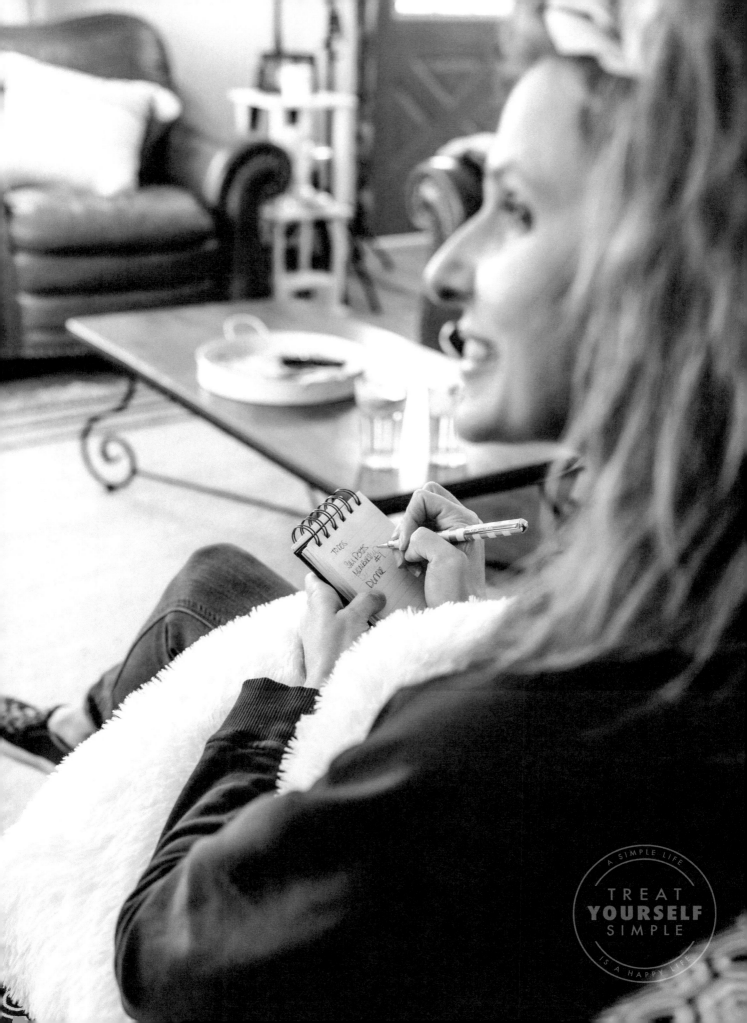

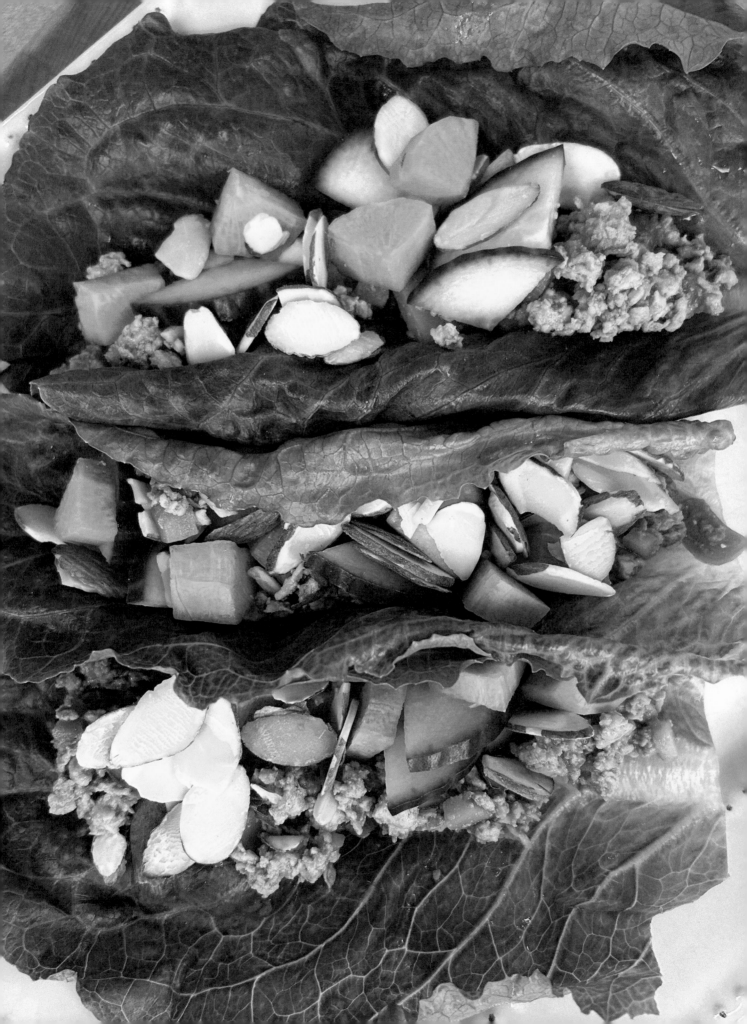

CHICKEN LETTUCE WRAPS STOVE

Serving Size:	2 servings	Cook time:	10 minutes
Prep time:	15 minutes	Needed:	Skillet, bowl, measuring cup, whisk, heat-safe spoon

DIRECTIONS

1 t ➤ Garlic, minced
½ T ➤ Ginger, fresh, peeled, minced or ¼ t ground Ginger
1 T ➤ Soy Sauce
1 T ➤ Rice Vinegar
¾ T ➤ Sesame Oil
½ T ➤ Honey
3 T ➤ Olive Oil

DRESSING

○ **Can make ahead. See Make Ahead Directions.** If not already prepared, combine the above ingredients in a small bowl or measuring cup. Whisk until well blended. Set dressing aside.

½ lb ➤ Chicken, ground
1 T ➤ Garlic, minced
½ T ➤ Ginger, fresh, peeled, minced or ¼ t ground Ginger

○ Heat skillet to medium-high. Add ground chicken; cook until browned through, about 5 minutes. Add above ingredients, cooking for about 1 minute, stir occasionally.

2 T ➤ Hoisin Sauce
1 T ➤ Rice Vinegar
1½ T ➤ Soy Sauce
½ T ➤ Pepper, red, crushed
½ t ➤ Sesame Oil

○ While the chicken is cooking, combine the above ingredients in a small bowl. Pour over the chicken mixture in the pan and stir well to combine.

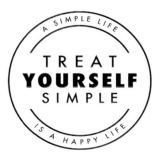

1 ➤ Onion, green, chopped
¼ C ➤ Water Chestnuts, diced

○ Add the above ingredients to skillet. Cook for about 2 minutes, stirring occasionally. Remove the skillet from the heat and set aside.

   ➤ Lettuce, butter or Romaine, wide leaf
½ C ➤ Carrots, shredded
½ C ➤ Cucumber halves, sliced
½ C ➤ Almonds, slivered
½ ➤ Avocado, large, diced

○ To make the wrap, fill each lettuce leaf with the chicken mixture and the above ingredients to use all ingredients. Drizzle with the sesame ginger dressing to taste. Divide into two plates. Serve immediately.

NOTES

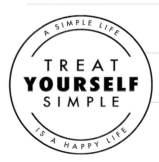

NOTES

TREAT
YOURSELF
SIMPLE

A SIMPLE LIFE

IS A HAPPY LIFE

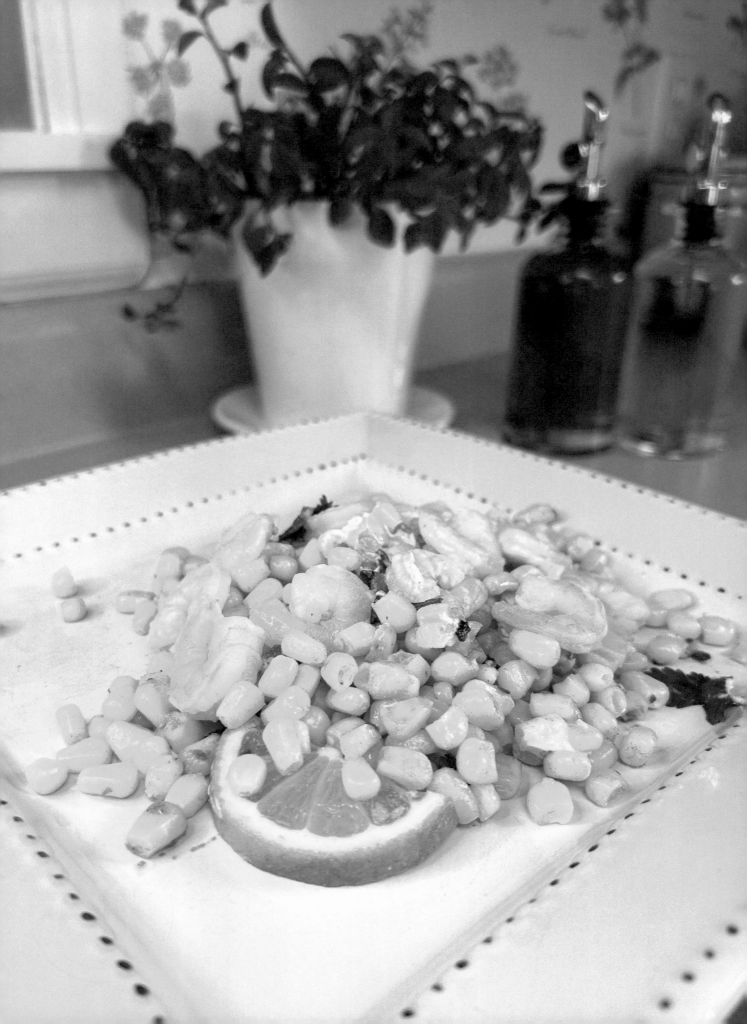

CILANTRO LIME SHRIMP GRILL OR OVEN

Serving Size:	2 servings	Cook time:	10 minutes
Prep time:	15 minutes	Needed:	Medium mixing bowl, spoon, foil, baking sheet, spatula

DIRECTIONS

○ Preheat grill on high or oven at 350° F.

dash ➤ Black Pepper, ground
1 T ➤ Cilantro, fresh, chopped
2 C ➤ Corn, frozen
½ t ➤ Pepper, red, crushed
1 t ➤ Cumin, ground
1½ t ➤ Garlic, minced
dash ➤ Kosher Salt
½ t ➤ Olive Oil
12 ➤ Shrimp, large, peeled and deveined or 2 C Salad Shrimp

○ In a medium mixing bowl, combine the above ingredients and toss together. Set aside.

1 T ➤ Butter
1 ➤ Lime, sliced into rounds

○ Lay out two pieces of foil, Place shrimp mixture on one piece of foil. Top with 1 T butter and lime slices. Place second piece of foil on top and seal pack.

GRILL

○ Place shrimp pack on grill.

OVEN

○ Place on baking sheet.

Grill/bake shrimp for 8–10 minutes or until shrimp is pink and eaches 165° F. Serve warm.

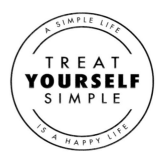

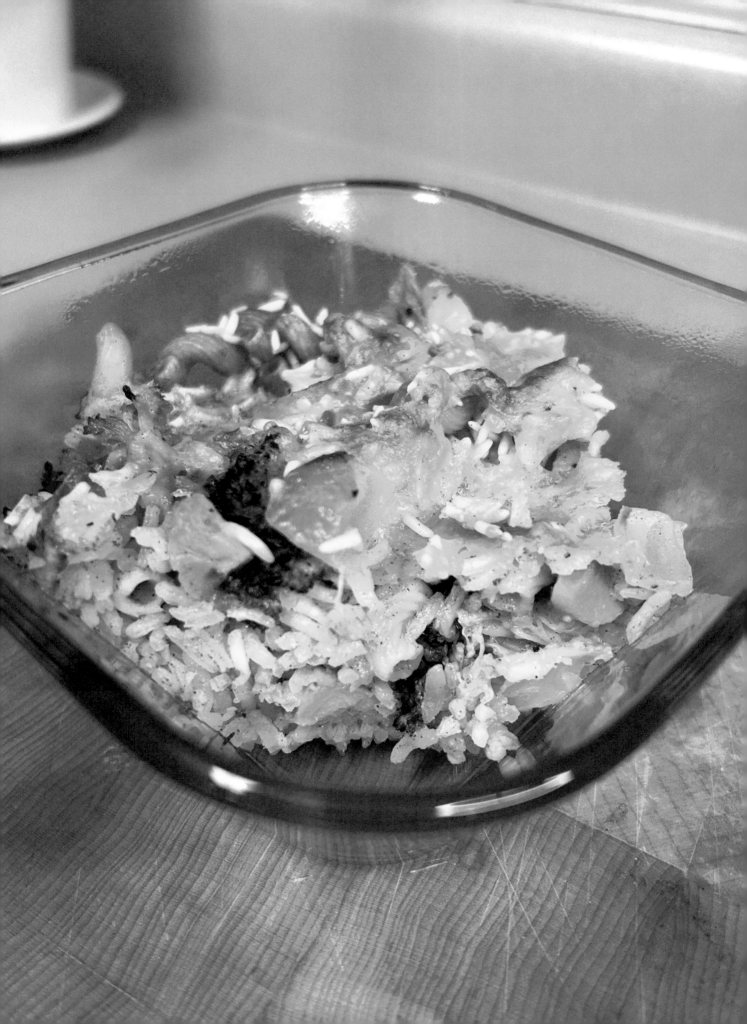

BROCCOLI CHEDDAR CHICKEN CASSEROLE 2/1   OVEN

Please note: Makes Chicken for Chicken Enchilada Stuffed Squash 2/1

Serving Size:	2 servings	**Cook time:**	1 hour 50 minutes
Prep time:	15 minutes	**Needed:**	Medium saucepan, heat-safe spoon, baking dish

DIRECTIONS

○ Preheat oven to 425º F.

Coat baking dish with cooking spray. Set aside.

½ T ➤ Olive Oil
½ C ➤ Onion, sweet, chopped
½ C ➤ Carrot, shredded

○ Heat medium saucepan over medium heat. Add rest of above ingredients, cooking for about 5 minutes or until fragrant.

4 ➤ Chicken Breasts, 4 oz each, cut into bite-sized pieces
dash ➤ Kosher Salt
dash ➤ Black Pepper, ground

○ Add chicken to same medium saucepan. Season with salt & pepper. Cook until golden brown, about 2–3 minutes for each side. Remove from heat. Set aside.

NOTE: *Set aside half of the chicken for* **Chicken Enchilada Stuffed Squash 2/1.** *Cool, and store in an airtight container. Refrigerate for 7–10 days.*

1 T ➤ Butter
1 C ➤ Rice, Jasmine,
2 oz ➤ Pasta, Orzo
1 T ➤ Thyme, fresh, chopped

○ Add above ingredients to already heated medium saucepan. Cook until golden and toasted, 2–3 minutes. Add chicken back to medium saucepan.

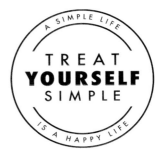

1½ C ➤ Broth, Chicken

○ Add the broth, bringing to a boil over high heat.

1½ C ➤ Broccoli florets, frozen
1 ➤ Bay leaf
¼ t ➤ Garlic Powder
¼ t ➤ Cayenne Pepper
dash ➤ Kosher Salt
dash ➤ Black Pepper, ground

○ Add the above ingredients to same medium saucepan.
Bring to a boil over high heat again, then cover and reduce heat to low.
Cook covered for 20–25 minutes until rice is mostly cooked.

1 T ➤ Lemon Juice
¼ C ➤ Milk

○ Add the above ingredients to saucepan, stir together,
then transfer the mixture to prepared casserole dish. Spread evenly.

¾ C ➤ Cheese, Cheddar, sharp, shredded

○ Sprinkle cheese over the top of the casserole. Bake 15-20 minutes
or until the cheese is melted and just beginning to brown. Serve warm.

NOTES

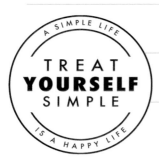

NOTES

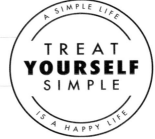

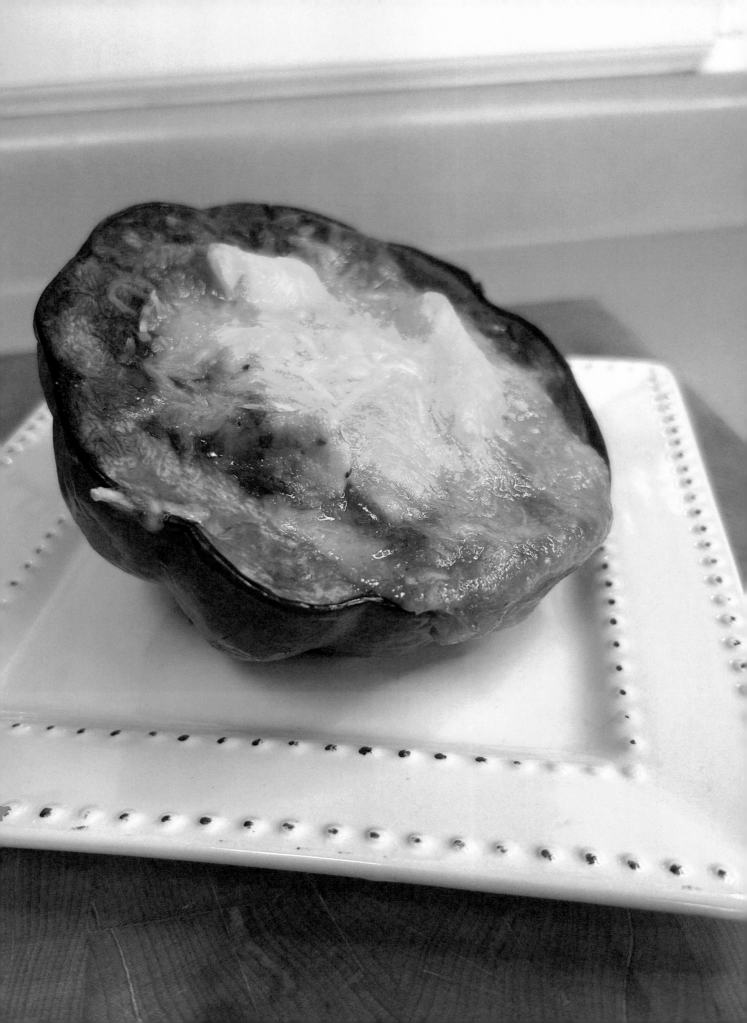

CHICKEN ENCHILADA STUFFED SQUASH 2/1 OVEN

Please note: Chicken was prepared from Broccoli Cheddar Chicken Casserole 2/1

Serving Size:	2 servings	Cook time:	22–55 minutes
Prep time:	10 minutes	Needed:	Two baking dishes, skillet, heat-safe spoon

DIRECTIONS

1 ⊳ Squash, Acorn, small, halved, seeds removed

SQUASH

○ **Can make ahead. See Make Ahead Directions.** If not already prepared, preheat oven to 425º F. Place squash in baking dish. Bake for 30 minutes until tender.

½ T ⊳ Olive Oil
2 T ⊳ Onions, sweet, fresh, chopped
1 t ⊳ Garlic, minced
¼ t ⊳ Cumin, ground
dash ⊳ Kosher Salt
dash ⊳ Black Pepper, ground

○ Coat skillet with olive oil over medium-high heat. Add above ingredients. Cook until slightly soften, about 2 minutes, stirring occasionally.

2 ⊳ Chicken Breasts, 4 oz each, cut into bite-sized pieces, from **Broccoli Cheddar Chicken Casserole 2/1**
½ can ⊳ Enchilada Sauce, red, 10 oz can

○ Add the above ingredient. Bring to a boil. Simmer and cook until the sauce slightly thickens, about 5 minutes.

¼ C ⊳ Cilantro, fresh, chopped
½ C ⊳ Cheese, Cheddar, shredded
optional ⊳ Sour Cream

○ Place squash halves cut side up in a baking dish. Divide the chicken filling evenly between the squash halves. Top with cilantro and cheese. Bake until cheese is lightly golden and melted, about 10–12 minutes. Top with sour cream and more cilantro. Serve warm.

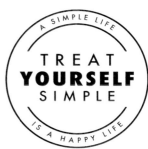

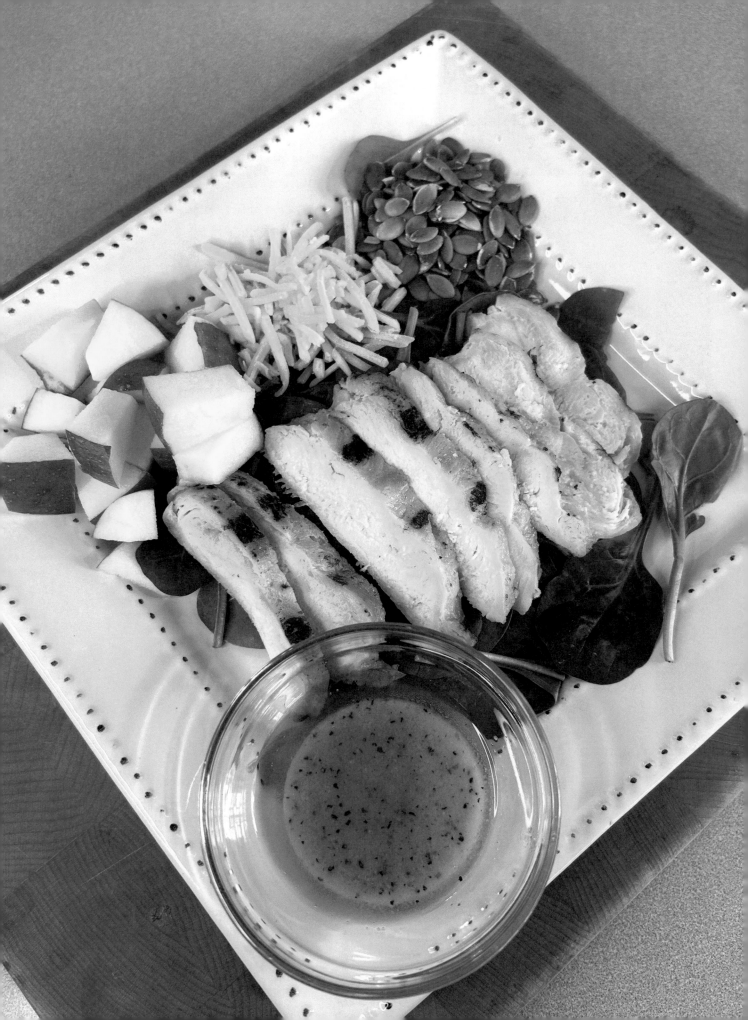

CHICKEN SPINACH SALAD STOVE

Serving Size:	2 servings	Cook time:	No cooking required
Prep time:	15 minutes	Needed:	Small bowl or measuring cup, medium mixing bowl, large spoon

DIRECTIONS

½ t ➤ Mustard, Dijon
½ t ➤ Honey
1 t ➤ Red Wine Vinegar
2 T ➤ Olive Oil
dash ➤ Kosher Salt
dash ➤ Black Pepper, ground

DRESSING

○ **Can make ahead. See Make Ahead Directions.** If not already prepared, Combine above ingredients in small bowl; whisk together until well blended; refrigerate until ready to serve.

2 ➤ Chicken Breasts. 4 oz each

○ Coat skillet with olive oil over medium-high heat. Add chicken, season with salt & pepper; cook for 8–12 minutes, flipping at least once until internal temperature reaches 165º F. Remove from heat. Slice chicken breasts into strips.

1 ➤ Apple, cubed
⅓ C ➤ Cheese, Cheddar, shredded
¼ C ➤ Pumpkin Seeds

○ Toss above ingredients in a medium bowl.

2 C ➤ Spinach

○ Divide spinach between two plates. Divide half of the prepared chicken strips on spinach on each plate. Add apple mixture on top of spinach. Top with dressing. Serve cold.

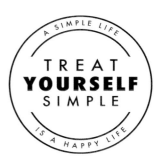

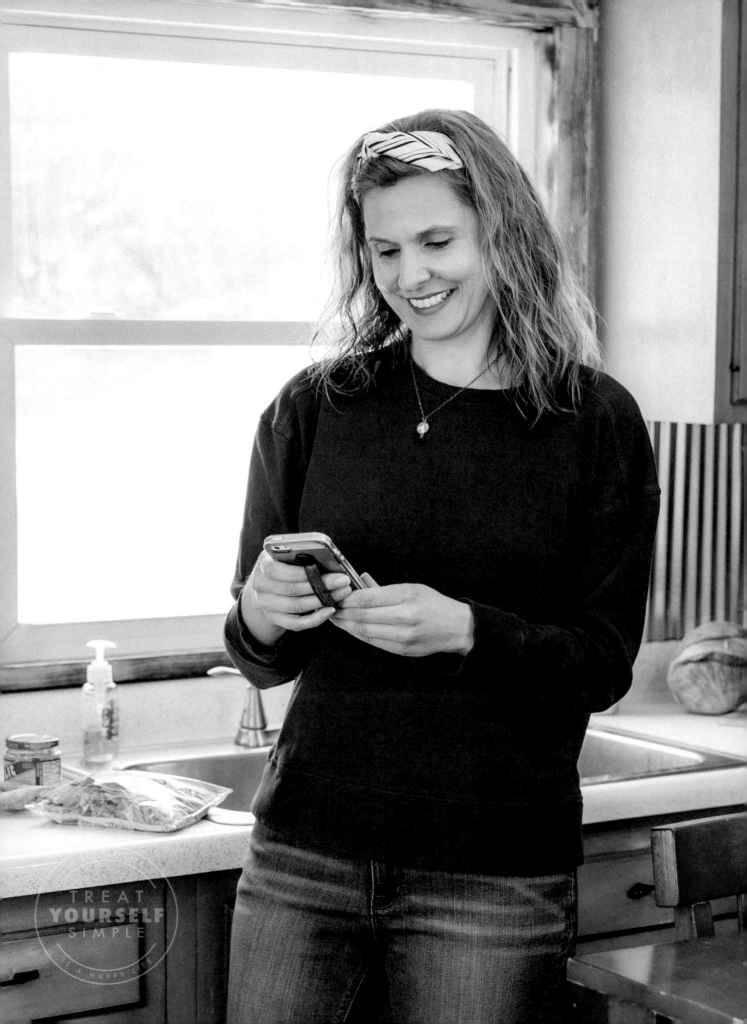

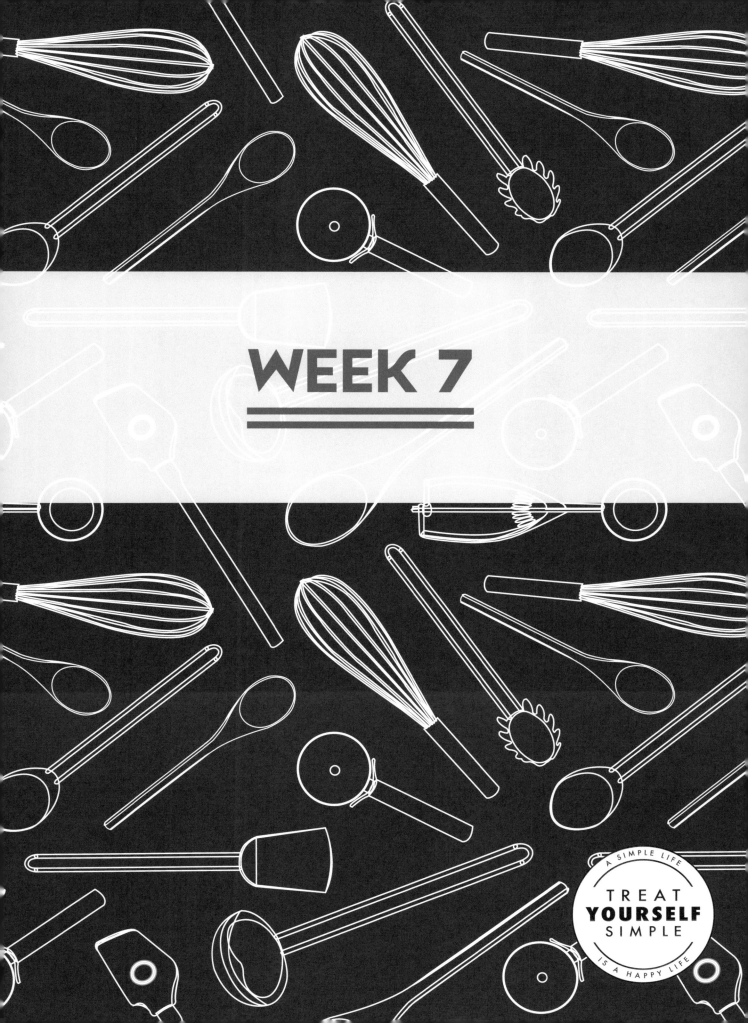

WEEK 7

WEEK 7 MENU PLAN

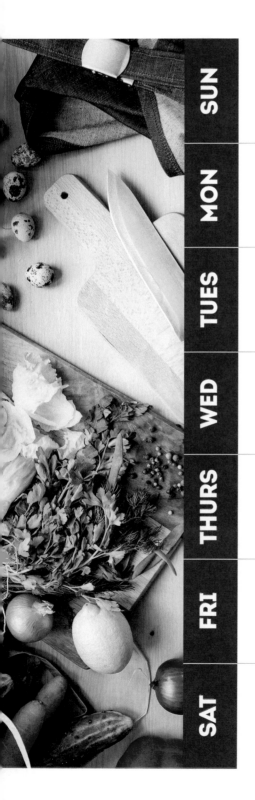

SUN

SWEET SPICY SALMON

Cottage Cheese
Pears

MON

HARVEST CHIPOTLE CHILI 2/1

Brussel Sprouts
Apple Slices

TUES

PUMPKIN FRENCH TOAST

Yogurt
Pomegranate Avrils

WED

STUFFED SQUASH WITH BEEF & FETA 2/1

Green Beans
Spiced Pears

THURS

FRENCH GREEN VEGETABLES AU GRATIN

Guacamole and Chips
Fresh Fruit Bowl

FRI

CREAMY SALMON LINGUINE

Fresh Salad
Orange Slices

SAT

HAM, CHEESE & SPINACH PUFFS

Sweet Potato Discs
Bananas

WEEK 7 GROCERY LIST

BY MEAL

SWEET SPICY SALMON

dash	Black Pepper, ground
dash	Kosher Salt
½ T	Mustard, Dijon
1 T	Mayonnaise
1 T	Maple Syrup
¼ t	Cayenne Pepper
2	Salmon Filets, 4 oz each

HARVEST CHIPOTLE CHILI 2/1

1	Apple, tart, medium, fresh, chopped
½ C	Broth, Chicken
1 T	Chili Powder
1 lb	Beef, ground, ½ lb for **Stuffed Squash with Beef & Feta 2/1**
1 T	Garlic, minced
¼ t	Kosher Salt
¼ C	Onion, sweet, fresh, chopped
1 T	Paprika, ground
¼	Bell Pepper, any color, chopped
½ C	Beans, pinto, 15 oz can, drained (you can also use kidney beans, black beans, or garbanzo beans)
½ can	Tomatoes, stewed, 15 oz can
1	Sweet Potato, cut into bite-sized pieces
¼ C	Corn, frozen

PUMPKIN FRENCH TOAST

⅓ C	Milk
¼ C	Pumpkin Pureé
2	Eggs, large
1 T	Maple Syrup
½ t	Vanilla Extract
½ t	Cinnamon, ground
dash	Nutmeg, ground
dash	Ginger, ground
4 slices	Bread
	Butter

STUFFED SQUASH WITH BEEF & FETA 2/1

2 slices	Bacon, crumbled or 2 T Real Bacon Bits/Crumbles
2 oz	Spinach, baby, fresh
dash	Black Pepper, ground
3 T + 1 t	Dill, fresh, chopped
1	Egg, lightly beaten
¼ C	Cheese, Feta, crumbled
1 t	Garlic, minced
½ lb	Beef, ground, from **Harvest Chipotle Chili 2/1**
¼ C	Rice, Jasmine, cooked (or Brown Rice, Quinoa, Barley or Farro)
dash	Kosher Salt
1	Squash, summer, chopped
1	Zucchini, chopped

FRENCH GREEN VEGETABLES AU GRATIN

½ T	Olive Oil
½ C	Onion, sweet, fresh, chopped
1 T	Flour
¾ C	Milk
¼ t	Poultry Seasoning
dash	Kosher Salt
dash	Black Pepper, ground
¾ C	Cheese, Colby Jack, shredded
1 C	Spinach, frozen, chopped
1 C	Broccoli, frozen
1	Zucchini, medium, fresh, chopped
1½ T	Butter
½ C	Breadcrumbs
2 T	Cheese, Parmesan, shredded

BY MEAL

CREAMY SALMON LINGUINE

1 t	Black Pepper, ground
1 T	Butter
½ C	Cheese, Parmesan, shredded
1 C	Cream, heavy whipping
1½ T	Basil, fresh, chopped
1½ t	Garlic, minced
1 t	Kosher Salt
1 T + 1 t	Lemon Juice
4 oz	Pasta, linguine
2	Salmon patties, 4 oz each, pre-made, frozen
½ C	Broccoli florets, frozen

HAM, CHEESE & SPINACH PUFFS

½ C	Spinach, baby, chopped
dash	Black Pepper, ground
½ T	Butter
½ T	Flour
2 T	Ham, cooked, diced
dash	Kosher Salt
¼ C	Milk
¼ C	Cheese, Mozzarella, shredded
1 sheet	Puff Pastry

WEEK 7 PREP

Mince 11 Garlic cloves ~ Harvest Chipotle Chili, Stuffed Squash with Beef & Feta 2/1, Creamy Salmon Linguine

Chop ¼ Bell Pepper, any color ~ Harvest Chipotle Chili

Chop ¾ Sweet Onion ~ Harvest Chipotle Chili 2/1, French Green Vegetables Au Gratin

Cut 1 Sweet Potato into bite-sized pieces ~ Harvest Chipotle Chili

Chop 1 Summer Squash ~ Stuffed Squash with Beef & Feta 2/1

Chop 2 Zucchinis ~ Stuffed Squash with Beef & Feta 2/1, French Green Vegetables Au Gratin

Shred ¾ C Colby Cheese ~ French Green Vegetables Au Gratin

Shred ¼ C Mozzarella Cheese ~ Ham Cheese and Spinach Puffs

WEEK 7 MAKE AHEAD

Prepare 2 slices Bacon ~ Stuffed Squash with Beef & Feta 2/1

Prepare ¼ C Jasmine Rice ~ Stuffed Squash with Beef & Feta 2/1

NOTES

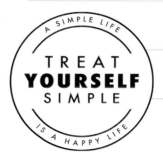

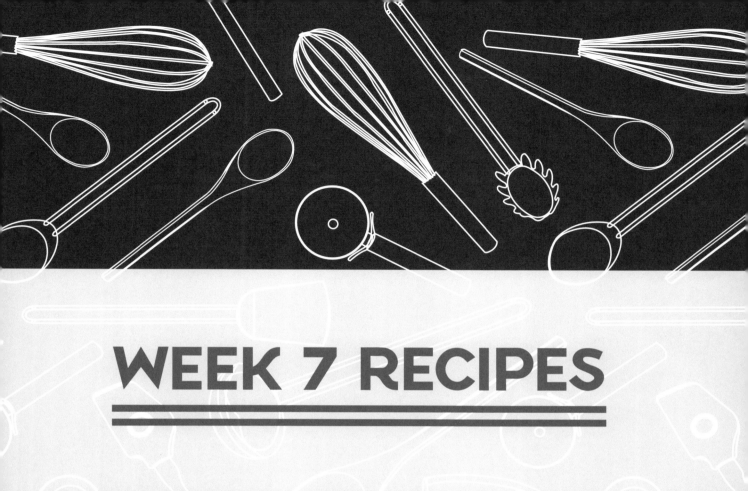

WEEK 7 RECIPES

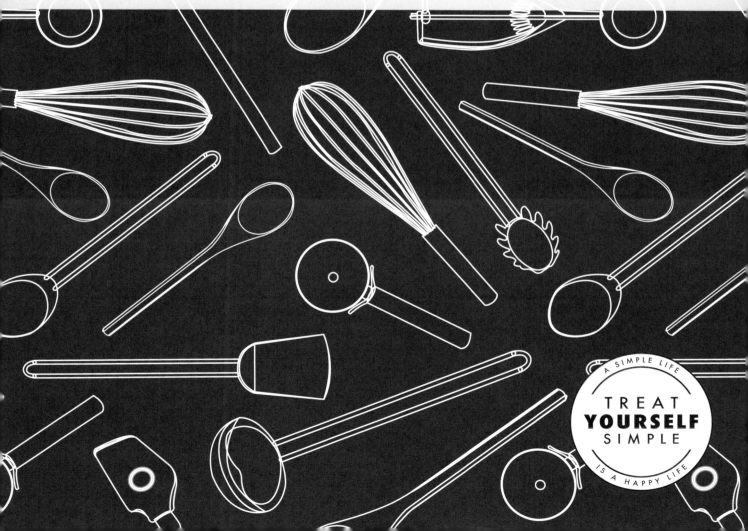

A SIMPLE LIFE
TREAT
YOURSELF
SIMPLE
IS A HAPPY LIFE

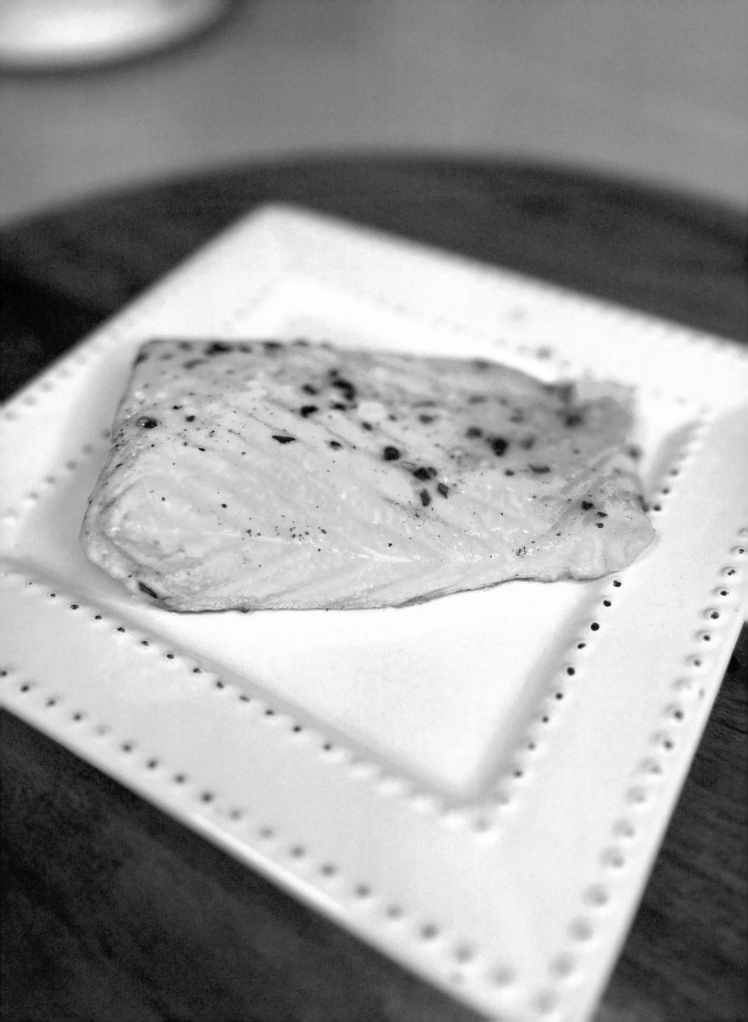

SWEET SPICY SALMON   GRILL OR OVEN

Serving Size:	2 servings	Cook time:	8–10 minutes
Prep time:	4 minutes	Needed:	Small bowl or measuring cup, spoon, foil, baking sheet, spatula

DIRECTIONS

○ Preheat oven to 400° F. Line baking sheet with aluminum foil. Set aside.

½ T ➢ Mustard, Dijon
1 T ➢ Mayonnaise
1 T ➢ Maple Syrup
¼ t ➢ Cayenne Pepper

○ To make the glaze, combine the above ingredients in a small bowl or measuring cup.

2 ➢ Salmon Filets, 4 oz
dash ➢ Kosher Salt
dash ➢ Black Pepper, ground

○ Place salmon pieces on the prepared baking sheet and sprinkle with kosher salt and black pepper. Slather the glaze on the salmon (tops and sides). Bake for 8 minutes or until the internal temperature is 145° F. Serve warm.

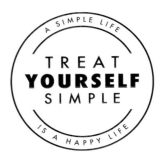

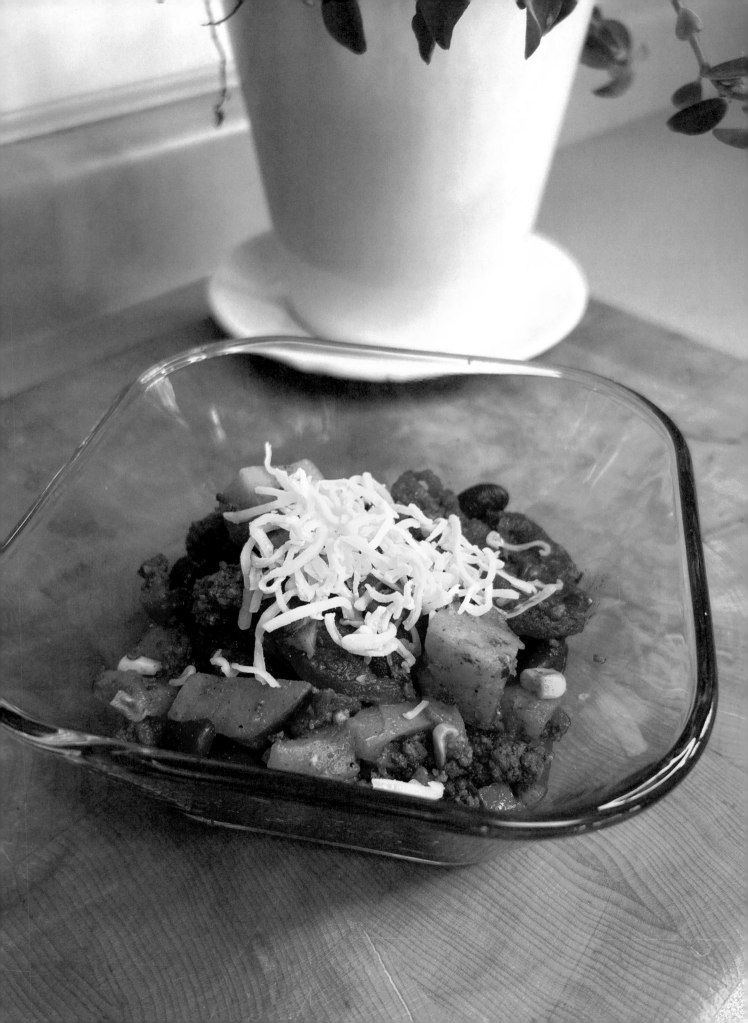

HARVEST CHIPOTLE CHILI 2/1 STOVE

Please note: Makes Ground Beef for Stuffed Squash with Beef & Feta 2/1

Serving Size:	2 servings	Cook time:	25 minutes
Prep time:	30 minutes	Needed:	Small bowl or measuring cup, skillet, heat-safe spoon

DIRECTIONS

¼ ➤ Bell Pepper, any color, chopped
1 T ➤ Paprika, ground
1 T ➤ Chili Powder
1 T ➤ Garlic, minced

○ Combine above ingredients in a small bowl or measuring cup. Set aside.

1 lb ➤ Beef, ground

○ **Can make ahead. See Make Ahead Directions.** If not already prepared, add ground beef in a skillet over medium to medium-high heat; cook until meat is browned. Break up the meat as it cooks. Drain off fat if needed.

NOTE: *Remove half of the ground beef for* **Stuffed Squash with Beef & Feta 2/1.** *Set aside, cool, and store in an airtight container. Refrigerate for 7–10 days.*

¼ C ➤ Onion, sweet, fresh, chopped

○ Add above ingredient to skillet with ground beef, cooking until onion is tender.

○ Add pepper mixture to ground beef/onion in skillet. Cook and stir for 5 minutes.

1 ➤ Sweet Potato, cut into bite-sized pieces
½ C ➤ Beans, pinto, 15 oz can, drained (you can also use kidney beans, black beans, or garbanzo beans)
¼ C ➤ Corn, frozen
½ C ➤ Tomatoes, stewed, 15 oz can, do not drain
½ C ➤ Broth, Chicken
1 ➤ Apple, tart, medium, fresh, chopped
¼ t ➤ Kosher Salt

○ Stir in the above ingredients. Bring to a boil and reduce heat. Simmer, covered for 25–30 minutes or until sweet potato is tender. Divide between two bowls.

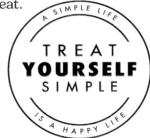

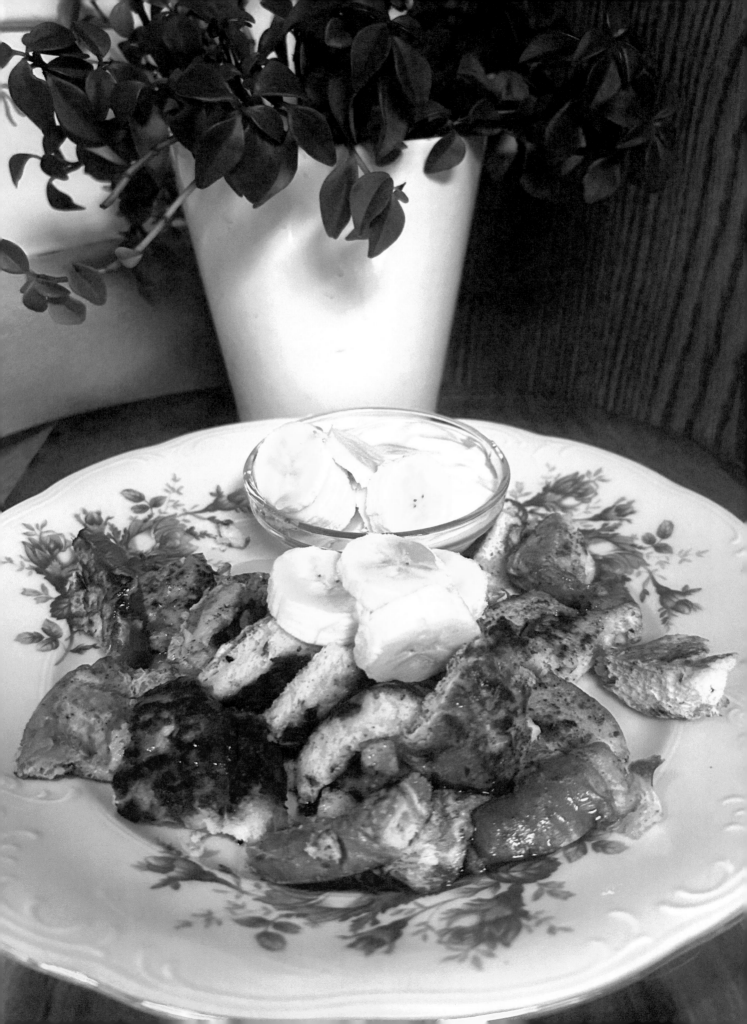

PUMPKIN FRENCH TOAST STOVE

Serving Size:	2 servings	Cook time:	15 minutes
Prep time:	15 minutes	Needed:	Mixing bowl, shallow dish, skillet or griddle, spatula

DIRECTIONS

○ Preheat skillet to medium heat or griddle to 350º F.

⅓ C ➤ Milk
¼ C ➤ Pumpkin Pureé
2 ➤ Eggs, large
1 T ➤ Maple Syrup
½ t ➤ Vanilla Extract
½ t ➤ Cinnamon, ground
dash ➤ Nutmeg
dash ➤ Ginger

○ Whisk together the above ingredientsIn in a mixing bowl until well combined. Pour into a shallow dish.

4 slices ➤ Bread
➤ Butter

○ Butter skillet and dip bread into egg mixture; allow a few seconds to absorb the egg mixture on one side. Flip over to opposite side.

○ Transfer to skillet or griddle and cook until golden brown on bottom, then lift, add more butter to skillet or griddle once more and flip French toast to opposite side and cook until golden brown. Serve warm with butter and maple syrup.

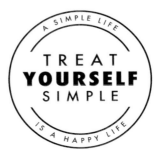

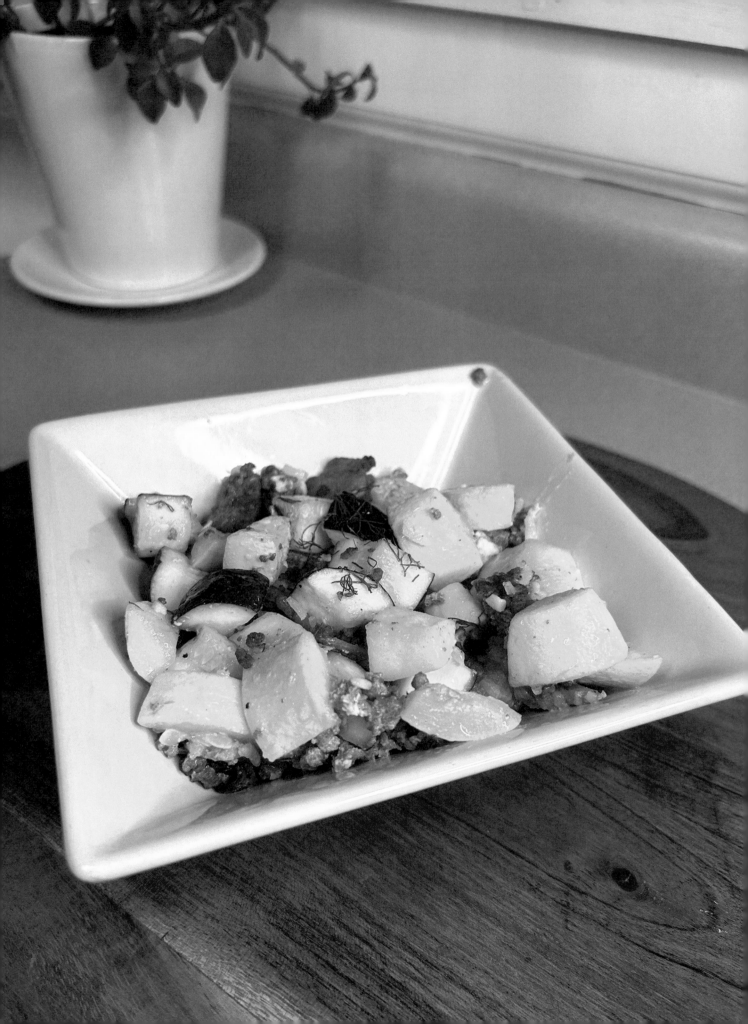

STUFFED SQUASH WITH BEEF & FETA 2/1 STOVE/OVEN

Please note: Ground Beef was prepared from Harvest Chipotle Chicken 2/1

Serving Size:	2 servings	Cook time:	40 minutes
Prep time:	20 minutes	Needed:	Skillet, medium saucepan, baking sheet, medium bowl, heat-safe spoon

DIRECTIONS

- ○ Preheat oven to 350° F

- ○ Coat baking sheet with cooking spray. Set aside.

2 slices ➤ Bacon, crumbled or 2 T Real Bacon Bits/Crumbles

- ○ **Can make ahead. See Make Ahead Directions.** If not already prepared, preheat oven to 375º F. Line baking sheet with aluminum foil.
Place bacon slices on baking sheet. Bake for 25 minutes.
Remove from oven and baking sheet. Line paper towels to a plate.
Place cooked bacon slices on paper towels to drain grease.
Let cool for about 5 minutes.

- ○ Crumble bacon or cut into small pieces with kitchen scissors.
Set aside to use for garnish. Refrigerate any extra for 7–10 days
and use for other meals.

¼ C ➤ Rice, Jasmine, cooked (or Brown Rice, Quinoa, Barley or Farro)

- ○ **Can make ahead. See Make Ahead Directions.** If not already prepared,
follow package directions, set aside.

½ lb ➤ Beef, ground, from **Harvest Chipotle Chili 2/1**
3 T ➤ Dill, fresh, chopped

- ○ Add above ingredients to skillet on medium heat, and cook,
stirring to combine, about 8–10 minutes

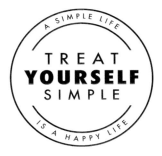

1 ➤ Squash, summer, chopped
1 ➤ Zucchini. chopped
dash ➤ Kosher Salt
1 t ➤ Garlic, minced

○ Add above ingredients to skillet, and cook, stirring occasionally, until tender, about 3 minutes.

2 oz ➤ Spinach, baby, fresh

○ Stir in above ingredient; cover and cook until spinach is wilted, about 2 minutes. Uncover and cook until liquid is almost evaporated, about 1 minute. Transfer beef mixture to a medium bowl; cool 10 minutes.

1 ➤ Egg, lightly beaten
dash ➤ Black Pepper, ground

○ Stir above ingredients plus prepared Jasmine rice into beef mixture.

¼ C ➤ Cheese, Feta, crumbled

○ Gently stir in above ingredient. Divide mixture into two servings, placing onto prepared baking sheet.

1 t ➤ Dill, fresh, chopped

○ Sprinkle with dill. Bake for 8–12 minutes until golden brown. Remove from heat. Serve warm.

NOTES

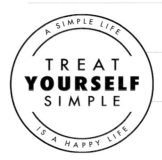

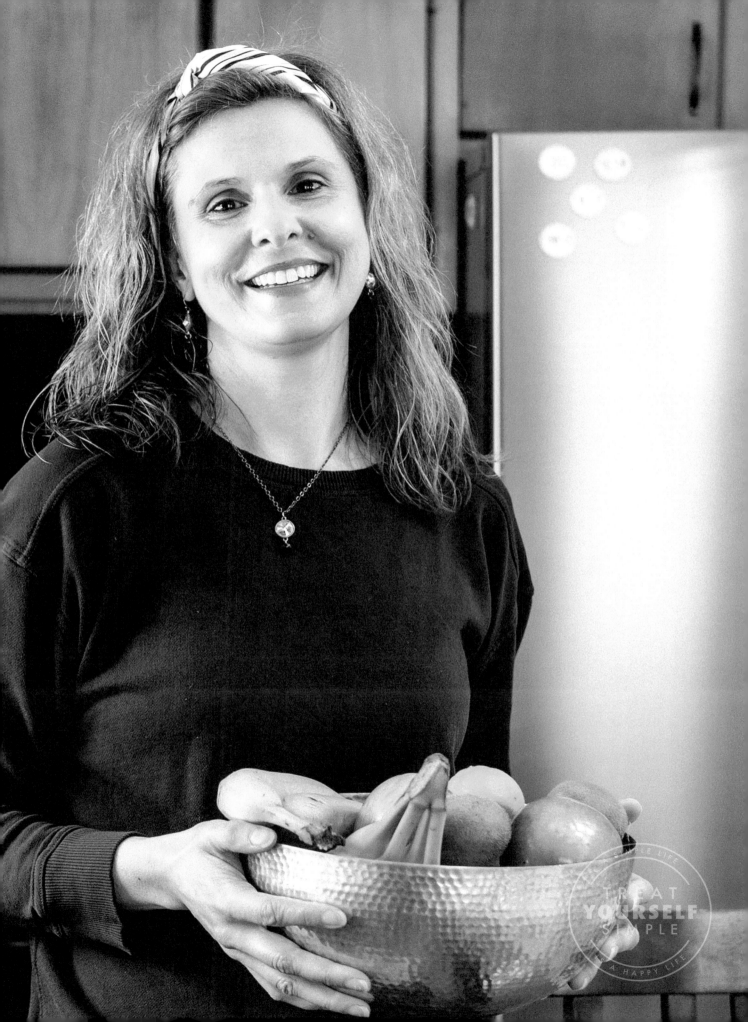

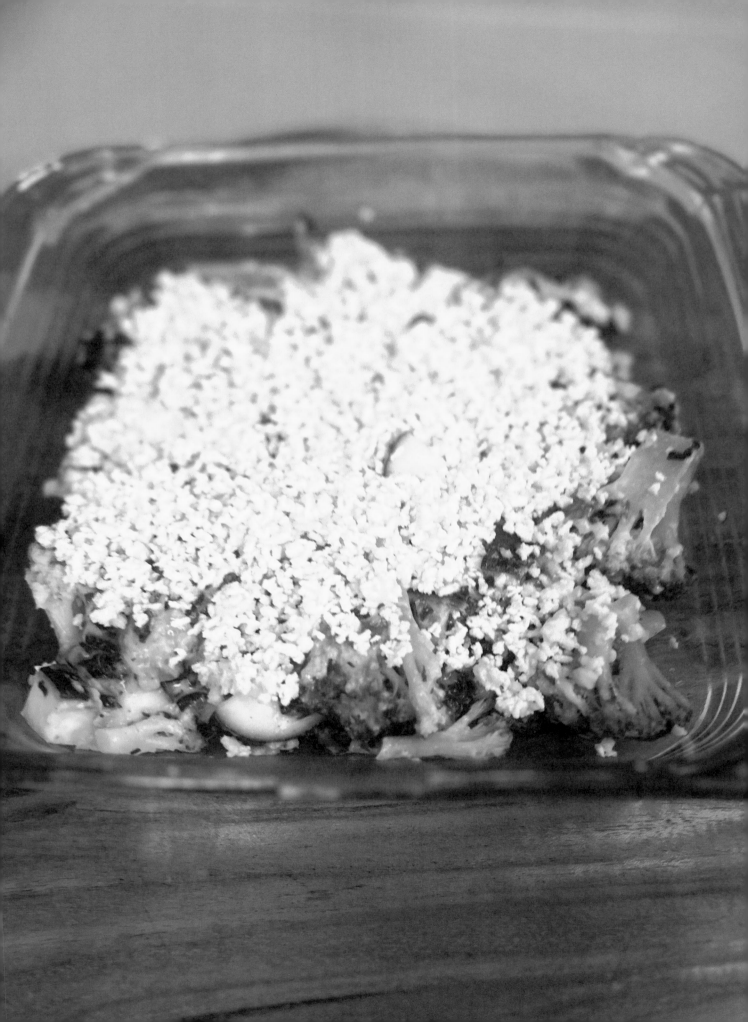

FRENCH GREEN VEGETABLES AU GRATIN OVEN

Serving Size:	2 servings	Cook time:	45 minutes
Prep time:	10 minutes	Needed:	Baking dish, skillet, measuring cup or small bowl, cooking spray, large pot, heat-safe spoon

DIRECTIONS

○ Preheat oven to 375° F. Spray a baking dish with cooking spray. Set aside.

½ T ➤ Olive Oil
½ C ➤ Onion, sweet, fresh, chopped

○ Coat skillet with olive oil over medium-high heat. Add onion, stir occasionally, about 5 minutes.

1 T ➤ Flour
¾ C ➤ Milk
¼ t ➤ Poultry Seasoning
dash ➤ Kosher Salt
dash ➤ Black Pepper, ground

○ Sprinkle flour over onions and continue to cook the mixture for 30 seconds. Add rest of above ingredients to the skillet. Stir constantly for 3–5 minutes until the sauce thickens.

¾ C ➤ Cheese, Colby Jack, shredded
1 C ➤ Spinach, frozen, chopped
1 C ➤ Broccoli, frozen
1 ➤ Zucchini, medium, fresh, chopped

○ Stir the above ingredients in same skillet; simmer for 2 minutes. Put in prepared baking dish.

1½ T ➤ Butter
½ C ➤ Breadcrumbs
2 T ➤ Cheese, Parmesan, shredded

○ Place butter in a glass measuring cup or small bowl; place in microwave; cook on high for 20 seconds. Stir in breadcrumbs and cheese. Sprinkle the mixture over the vegetable mixture. Bake for 30–40 minutes until breadcrumbs have turned golden brown. Serve warm.

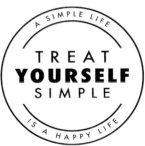

A SIMPLE LIFE
TREAT
YOURSELF
SIMPLE
IS A HAPPY LIFE

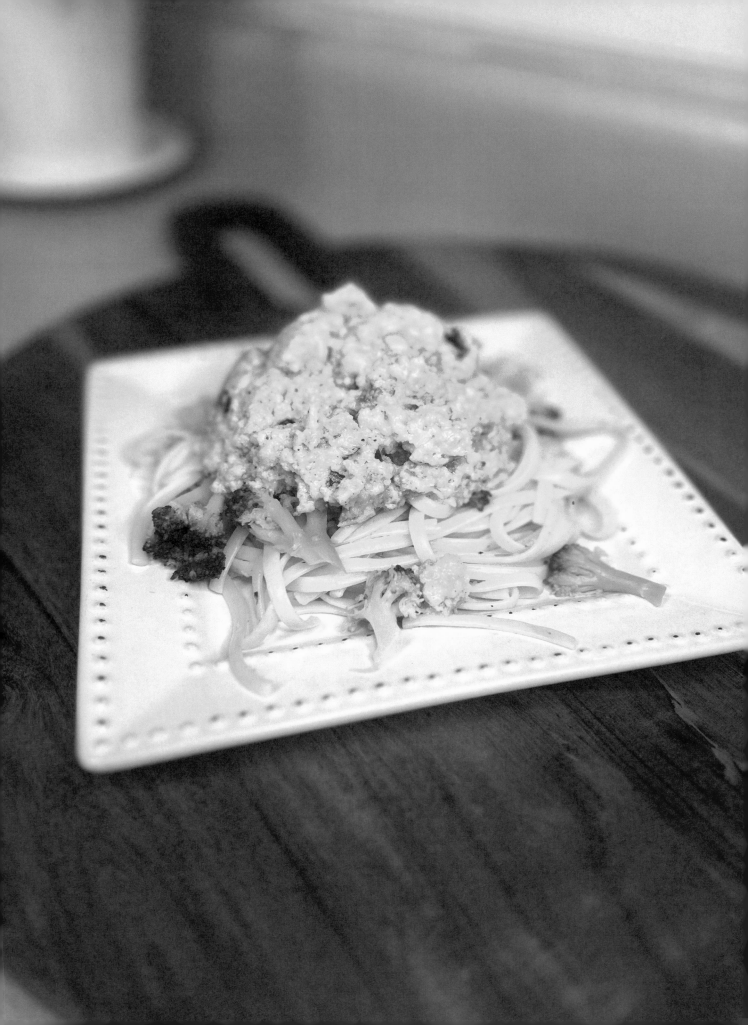

CREAMY SALMON LINGUINE STOVE

Serving Size:	2 servings	Cook time:	10 minutes
Prep time:	15 minutes	Needed:	Medium saucepan, skillet, colander, heat-safe spoon

DIRECTIONS

4 oz ➤ Pasta, linguine
½ C ➤ Broccoli florets, frozen

○ Cook linguine according to package directions, adding broccoli during the last 5 minutes of cooking. Drain. Set aside.

1 T ➤ Butter
1½ t ➤ Garlic, minced
1 C ➤ Cream, heavy whipping
1 T ➤ Lemon Juice

○ Meanwhile in a large skillet, heat butter over medium heat. Add garlic and cook, stirring for 1 minute. Stir in cream and lemon juice. Bring to a boil. Reduce heat and simmer uncovered, 2–3 minutes or until slightly thickened, stirring constantly.

2 ➤ Salmon patties, 4 oz each, pre-made, frozen
1 t ➤ Kosher Salt
1 t ➤ Black Pepper, ground

○ Add above ingredients; stir to blend; cook for about 2–3 minutes stirring occasionally.

½ C ➤ Cheese, Parmesan, shredded
1½ T ➤ Basil, fresh, chopped
1 t ➤ Lemon Juice

○ Stir in the above ingredients to the skillet. Serve immediately.

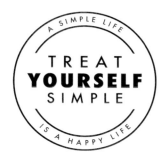
A SIMPLE LIFE
TREAT
YOURSELF
SIMPLE
IS A HAPPY LIFE

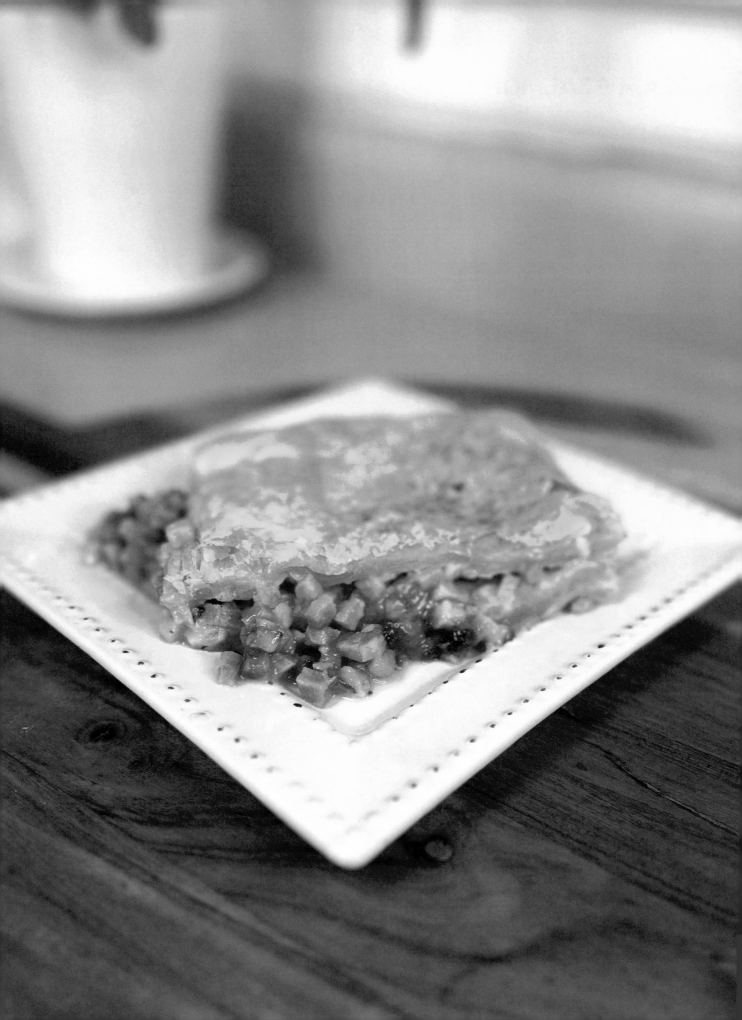

HAM, CHEESE & SPINACH PUFFS OVEN

Serving Size:	2 servings	Cook time:	40 minutes
Prep time:	15 minutes	Needed:	Baking sheet, medium saucepan, heat-safe spoon, spatula

DIRECTIONS

1 sheet ➤ Puff Pastry

○ Cut the puff pastry sheet in half; cut each half in half; will have four pieces; set aside in the refrigerator.

○ Preheat oven to 400° F.

○ Line baking sheet with parchment paper.

½ T ➤ Butter
½ T ➤ Flour
dash ➤ Kosher Salt
dash ➤ Black Pepper, ground

○ Melt butter over medium heat in a skillet. Add above ingredients. Cook, stirring frequently until the mixture becomes pale golden with a slightly nutty aroma, about 2 minutes

¼ C ➤ Milk

○ Pour in above ingredient, stirring constantly with a wooden spoon and whisk until smooth. Cook the mixture stirring constantly along the bottom of the skillet until boiling, about 7 minutes. Reduce heat to low. Simmer gently until sauce thickens, about 5 minutes.

½ C ➤ Spinach, baby, chopped
2 T ➤ Ham, cooked, diced

○ Add above ingredients and cook for 1 minute, stirring well. Remove from heat.

¼ C ➤ Cheese, Mozzarella, shredded

○ Arrange two pieces of puff pastry on prepared baking sheet. Divide mixture between the two pieces of puff pastry. Top with cheese. Place each of the remaining two pieces of puff pastry on top of the mixture. Bake for 20-25 minutes. Serve immediately.

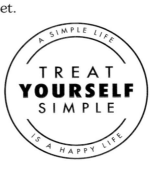

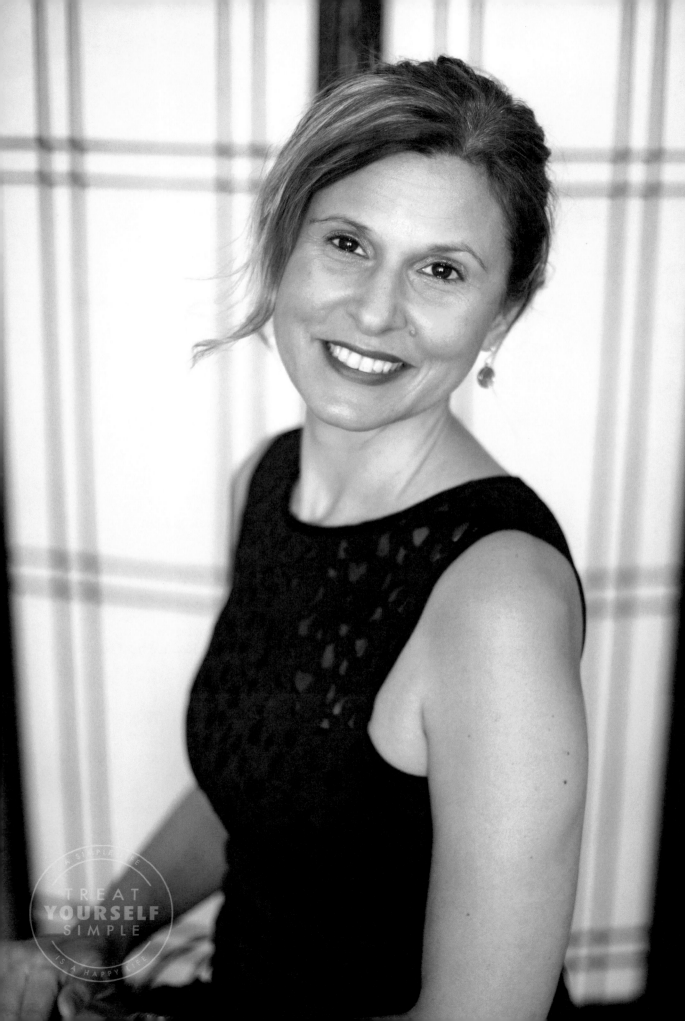

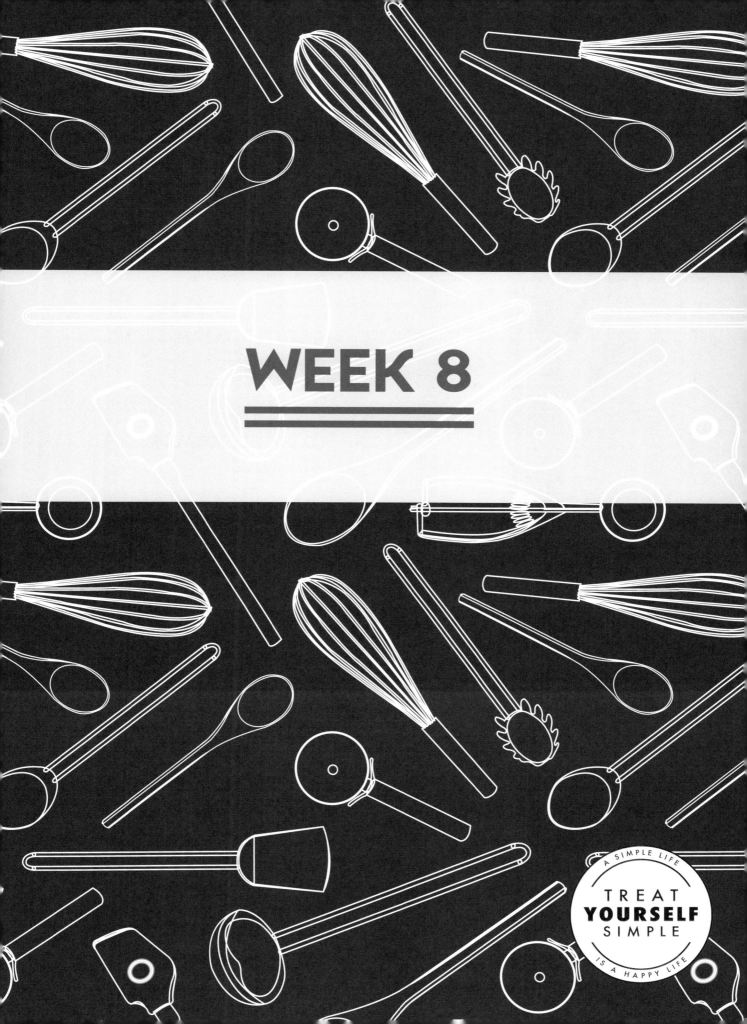

WEEK 8

WEEK 8 MENU PLAN

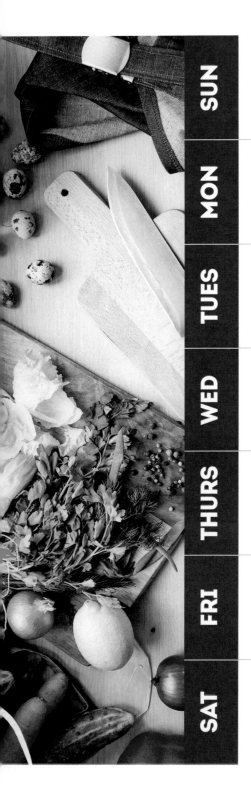

SUN

THAI COCONUT CHICKEN

Pomegranate Arils
Fresh Fruit Bowl

MON

APPLE CRANBERRY WALNUT SALAD

Vanilla Yogurt
Cinnamon Sliced Bananas

TUES

TACO STUFFED SWEET POTATOES 2/1

Fresh Salad
Garlic Toast

WED

PEAR, RASPBERRY & PISTACHIO SALAD

Cornbread
Cottage Cheese

THURS

ITALIAN SAUSAGE SPAGHETTI

Broccoli
Cinnamon Sliced Bananas

FRI

TEX MEX PULLED CHICKEN TACOS

Fresh Salad
Cinnamon Apples

SAT

ENCHILADA CASSEROLE 2/1

Broccoli
Coleslaw

WEEK 8 GROCERY LIST

BY MEAL

THAI COCONUT CHICKEN

¼ t	Black Pepper, ground
2	Chicken Breasts, 4 oz each
¼ C	Coconut Flakes
½ t	Coriander
1 t	Cumin, ground
½ t	Curry Powder
¼ t	Garlic Powder
¼ C	Greek Yogurt, plain
½ t	Kosher Salt
1 T	Lime Juice
2 T	Soy Sauce
2 T	Maple Syrup

APPLE CRANBERRY WALNUT SALAD

½	Apple, green, chopped
½	Apple, red, chopped
2 T	Apple Cider Vinegar
3 T	Apple Juice
3 C	Spinach, baby, fresh
⅛ t	Black Pepper, ground
2 T	Cheese, Feta, crumbed
2 T	Cranberries, dried
1 T	Honey
2 T	Olive Oil
¼ t	Kosher Salt
½ C	Walnuts

TACO STUFFED SWEET POTATOES 2/1

2	Sweet Potatoes, medium, 12–14 oz
1 lb	Beef, ground, ½ lb for **Enchilada Casserole 2/1**
1 C	Onion, sweet, chopped
½ t	Garlic, minced
optional	Cheese, Mexican, shredded
optional	Tomato, diced
optional	Avocado, diced or Guacamole
optional	Sour Cream
1 T	Taco Seasoning
½ C	Salsa, chunky
¼ C	Water

PEAR, RASPBERRY & PISTACHIO SALAD

2 t	Apple Cider Vinegar
¼ C	Cheese, Feta, crumbled
1 t	Chia Seeds
1½ T	Honey
2 C	Lettuce, Romaine, chopped
2 T	Mayonnaise
2 T	Milk
1	Pear, thinly sliced
¼ C	Pistachios, shelled
½ C	Raspberries, fresh

ITALIAN SAUSAGE SPAGHETTI

3 oz	Arugula, fresh
2–4 T	Cheese, Parmesan, shredded
½ lb	Italian Sausage, ground
1 t	Garlic, minced
dash	Kosher Salt
2 T	Lemon Juice
2 t	Olive Oil
¼ C	Pasta cooking water
4 oz	Pasta, spaghetti noodles

TEX MEX PULLED CHICKEN TACOS

1	Bell Pepper, any color, sliced
dash	Black Pepper, ground
¼ C	Cheese, Mexican, shredded
2	Chicken Breasts, 4 oz each, shredded
½ t	Chili Powder
¼ t	Cumin, ground
	Cilantro, fresh, chopped
1	Pepper, Jalapeno, halved, seeded
dash	Kosher Salt
1	Lime, cut into wedges
1 T	Olive Oil
½	Onion, sweet, fresh, cut into wedges
½ t	Oregano, dried
¼ C	Salsa
¼ C	Sour Cream
1	Tomato, medium, fresh, quartered
4	Tortilla Shells, 6–8", Flour or Corn

ENCHILADA CASSEROLE 2/1

¼ can	Beans, black, rinsed and drained, 15 oz can or ½ C
⅓ C	Cheese, Mexican, shredded
dash	Cumin, ground
½ lb	Beef, ground, browned, from **Taco Stuffed Sweet Potatoes 2/1**
to taste	Cilantro, fresh, chopped
⅓ C	Lettuce, shredded
¼	Onion, sweet, chopped
1 t	Salad Dressing, Italian
½ C	Salsa
¼ C	Sour Cream
½ T	Taco Seasoning
⅓ C	Tomato, fresh, medium, chopped
2	Tortilla Shells, 6–8", Flour or Corn

WEEK 8 PREP

Mince 3 Garlic Cloves ~ Italian Sausage Spaghetti, Taco Stuffed Sweet Potatoes 2/1

Slice 1 Bell Pepper, any color ~ Tex Mex Pulled Chicken Tacos

Chop 1¼ Sweet Onions ~ Taco Stuffed Sweet Potatoes 2/1, Enchilada Casserole 2/1

Chop ½ Sweet Onion into wedges ~ Tex Mex Pulled Chicken Tacos

Shred ¾ C Mexican Cheese ~ Tex Mex Pulled Chicken Tacos, Enchilada Casserole 2/1

WEEK 8 MAKE AHEAD

Prepare Marinade ~ Thai Coconut Chicken

Bake 2 Sweet Potatoes ~ Taco Stuffed Sweet Potatoes 2/1

Brown Italian Sausage ~ Italian Sausage Spaghetti

Taco Seasoning ~ Taco Stuffed Sweet Potatoes 2/1, Enchilada Casserole 2/1

Make Dressing ~ Apple Cranberry Walnut Salad, Pear Raspberry & Pistachio Salad

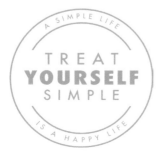

WEEK 8 RECIPES

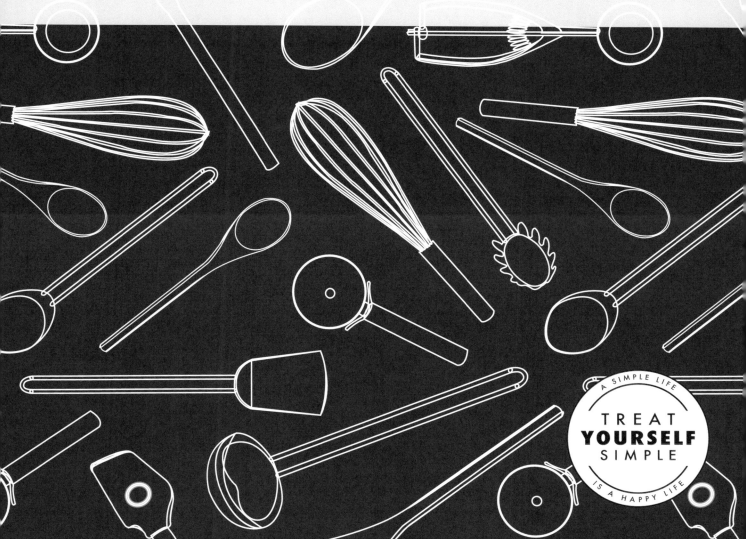

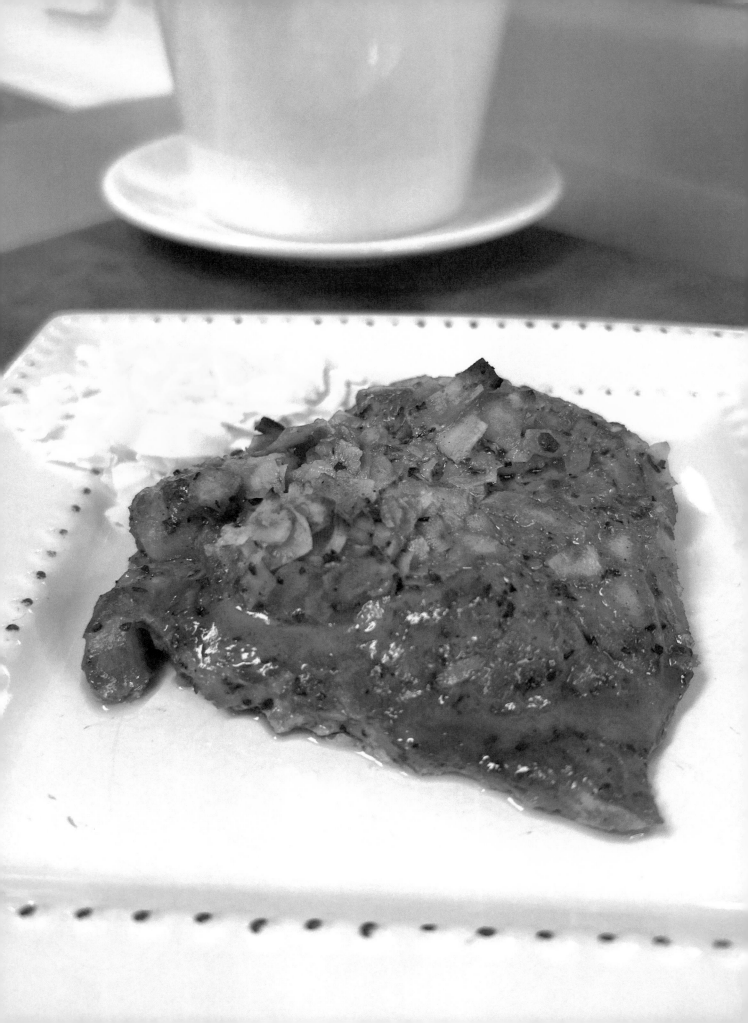

THAI COCONUT CHICKEN OVEN

Serving Size:	2 servings	Cook time:	8 minutes
Prep time:	10 minutes	Needed:	Zip top bag, baking sheet, spatula

2	➤	Chicken Breasts, 4 oz
¼ C	➤	Greek Yogurt, plain
¼ C	➤	Coconut Flakes
2 T	➤	Soy Sauce
2 T	➤	Maple Syrup
½ t	➤	Curry Powder
1 t	➤	Cumin, ground
½ t	➤	Coriander
½ t	➤	Kosher Salt
¼ t	➤	Black Pepper, ground
¼ t	➤	Garlic Powder
1 T	➤	Lime Juice

DIRECTIONS

MARINADE

○ **Can make ahead. See Make Ahead Directions.** If not already prepared, add above ingredients to a zip top bag and close the bag.
Use your hands to squish and mix everything until the chicken is coated.
Let refrigerate and marinate for at least 8 hours or overnight.

○ Preheat oven to 400º F. Place seasoned chicken on foil-lined baking sheet, dump rest of sauce over chicken. Bake for 20 minutes until desired doneness or internal temperature reaches 165º F. Remove from heat.
Divide chicken on two plates, serve warm.

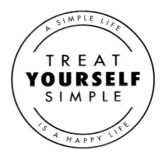

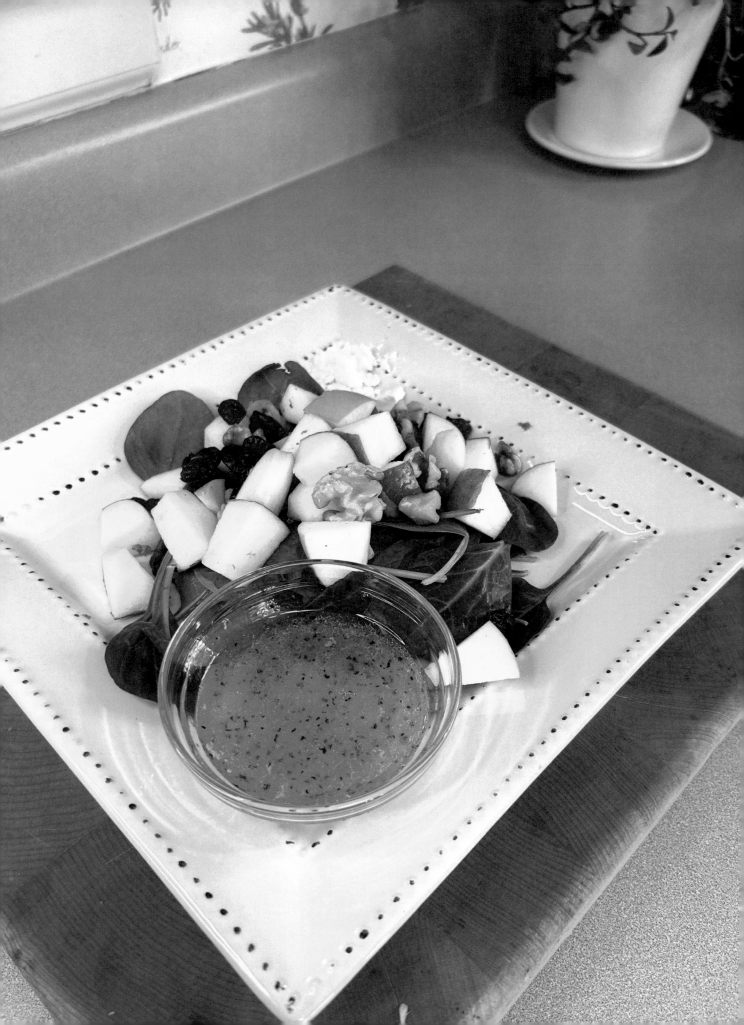

APPLE CRANBERRY WALNUT SALAD   NO COOK

Serving Size:	2 servings	Cook time:	No cooking required
Prep time:	15 minutes	Needed:	Medium bowl, measuring cup or small bowl, spoon

DIRECTIONS

3 T ➤ Apple Juice
2 T ➤ Apple Cider Vinegar
1 T ➤ Honey
¼ t ➤ Kosher Salt
⅛ t ➤ Black Pepper, ground
2 T ➤ Olive Oil

DRESSING

○ **Can make ahead. See Make Ahead Directions..** If not already prepared, Whisk above ingredients together in measuring cup or small bowl. Set aside in fridge.

½ ➤ Apple, red, chopped
½ ➤ Apple, green, chopped
½ C ➤ Walnuts
2 T ➤ Cheese, Feta, crumbled
2 T ➤ Cranberries, dried

○ Combine the above ingredients together in a medium bowl.

3 C ➤ Spinach, baby, fresh

○ Divide spinach between two plates; Top spinach with fruit & nut mixture; drizzle dressing over salad. Serve cold.

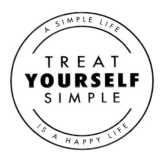

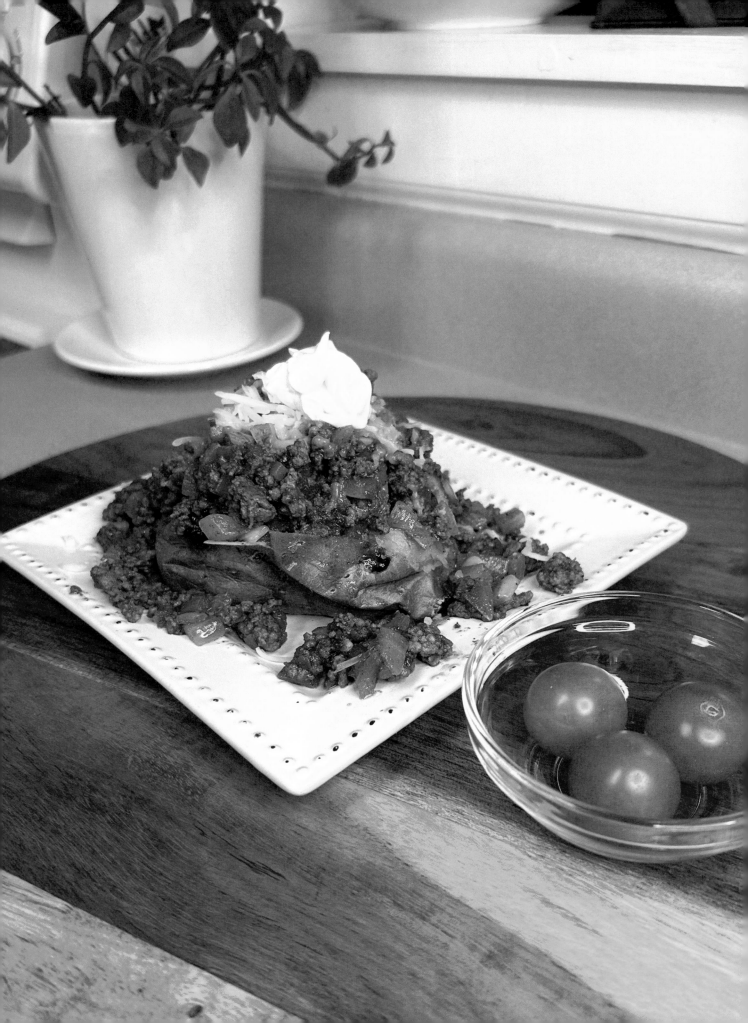

TACO STUFFED SWEET POTATOES 2/1   OVEN

Please note: Makes Ground Beef for Enchilada Casserole 2/1

Serving Size:	2 servings	Cook time:	45 minutes
Prep time:	5 minutes	Needed:	Baking dish, large skillet, heat-safe spoon

DIRECTIONS

○ Preheat oven to 400° F. Coat baking dish with olive oil. Set aside.

2 ➤ Sweet Potatoes, medium, 12–14 oz

○ **Can make ahead. See Make Ahead Directions.** If not already prepared, clean potatoes with water, dry completely, poke the potato 3–5 times all over, place in prepared baking dish, bake for approximately 45 minutes until tender to touch.

1 lb ➤ Beef, ground

○ Brown ground beef in a large skillet over medium-high heat.

1 C ➤ Onion, sweet, chopped
½ t ➤ Garlic, minced

○ **Can make ahead. See Make Ahead Directions.** If not already prepared, add above ingredients to ground beef in skillet. Cook for about 5 minutes until onion begins to soften.

NOTE: *Remove half of the ground beef for* **Enchilada Casserole 2/1.** *Set aside, cool, and store in an airtight container. Refrigerate for 7–10 days.*

1 T ➤ Taco Seasoning
½ C ➤ Salsa, chunky
¼ C ➤ Water

○ Add the taco seasoning and salsa. Reduce heat to medium-low and cook for about 5 more minutes until mixture has thickened and is heated through. Add up to ¼ cup of water to achieve desired consistency.

NOTE: *If ground beef mixture is already browned, add mixture to a skillet on medium-heat and then follow above directions.*

optional ➤ Cheese, Mexican, shredded
optional ➤ Tomato, diced
optional ➤ Avocado, diced or Guacamole
optional ➤ Sour Cream

○ Spoon the cooked taco meat over the sweet potatoes and add desired toppings such as shredded cheese, diced tomato, avocado, guacamole, or sour cream. Serve warm.

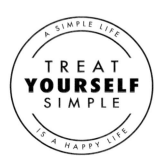

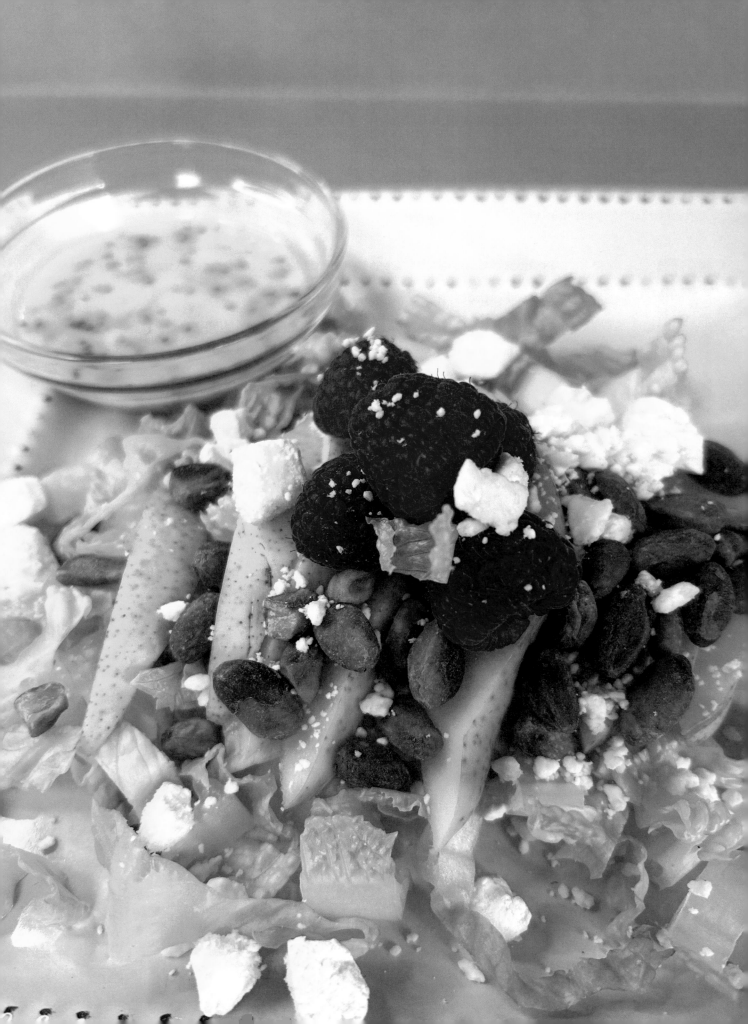

PEAR, RASPBERRY & PISTACHIO SALAD   NO COOK

Serving Size:	2 servings	Cook time:	No cooking required
Prep time:	15 minutes	Needed:	Measuring cup or small bowl, large bowl, spoon

DIRECTIONS

2 T ➤ Mayonnaise
2 T ➤ Milk
1½ T ➤ Honey
2 t ➤ Apple Cider Vinegar
1 t ➤ Chia Seeds

○ **Can make ahead. See Make Ahead Directions.** If not already prepared, Add the above ingredients in small bowl; whisk together until well blended; refrigerate until ready to serve.

2 C ➤ Lettuce, Romaine, chopped
½ C ➤ Raspberries, fresh
1 ➤ Pear, thinly sliced
¼ C ➤ Pistachios, shelled
¼ C ➤ Cheese, Feta, crumbled

○ Add the above ingredients to large bowl; toss together.
Add prepared dressing to salad mixture; toss to coat all of the ingredients.
Divide between two plates. Serve cold.

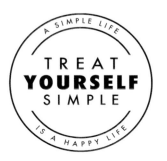

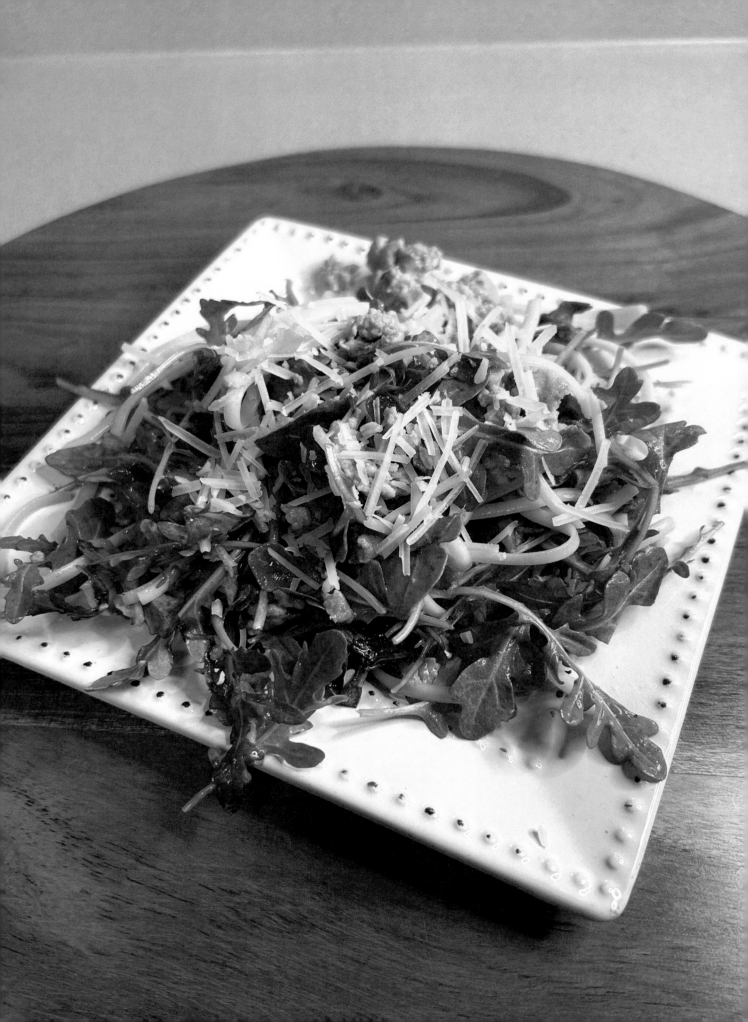

ITALIAN SAUSAGE SPAGHETTI STOVE

Serving Size:	2 servings	**Cook time:**	30–35 minutes
Prep time:	25 minutes	**Needed:**	Skillet, large bowl, colander, medium saucepan, heat-safe spoon

DIRECTIONS

½ lb ➤ Italian Sausage, ground
2 t ➤ Olive Oil

○ **Can make ahead. See Make Ahead Directions.** If not already prepared, coat skillet with olive oil over medium heat, add sausage to pan and brown well, breaking up into small pieces as it cooks.

4 oz ➤ Pasta, spaghetti noodles
dash ➤ Kosher Salt

○ If sausage is cooking, bring a medium saucepan of salted water to boil. Add spaghetti and cook 5–7 minutes, or until barely done and still al dente. Remove from heat. Set aside.

3 oz ➤ Arugula, fresh

○ Put arugula into a large bowl. When sausage is well browned, drain.

NOTE: *If pork mixture is already browned, add mixture to a skillet on medium heat to slightly warm mixture.*

○ Pour heated sausage over arugula. Add back to skillet and turn heat to very low.

1 t ➤ Garlic, minced

○ Add above ingredient and saute for 30 seconds.

¼ C ➤ Pasta cooking water
2 T ➤ Lemon Juice

○ Add above ingredients. Heat for 2 minutes. Let sit 2 minutes to wilt arugula.

REMEMBER: *When the noodles are done, scoop out another ¼ C of pasta cooking water in case you need it, then drain pasta well and put in the bowl with the arugula and sausage. If too dry, add a little lemon juice mixture until desired moistness is reached.*

2-4 T ➤ Cheese, Parmesan, shredded

○ Toss all the ingredients together. Divide into two servings. Serve hot with Parmesan cheese over top. Serve warm.

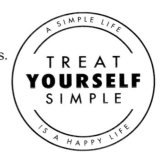

A SIMPLE LIFE
TREAT
YOURSELF
SIMPLE
IS A HAPPY LIFE

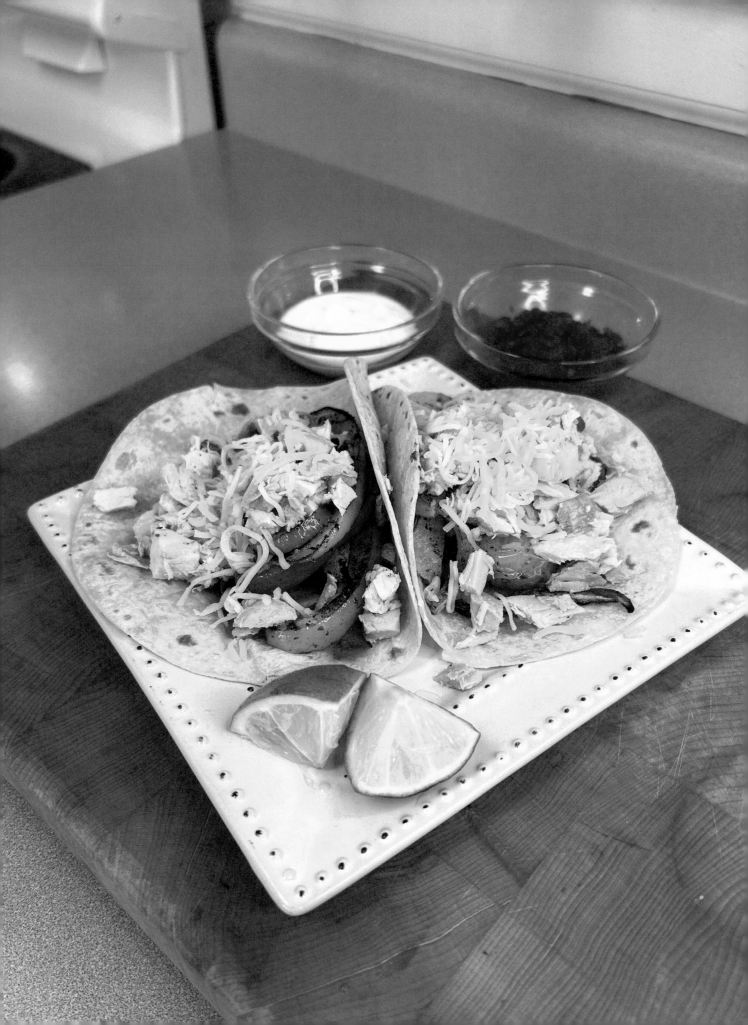

TEX MEX PULLED CHICKEN TACOS   OVEN

Serving Size:	2 servings	Cook time:	10 minutes
Prep time:	10 minutes	Needed:	Baking sheet, small bowl, spoon, two forks

DIRECTIONS

○ Preheat broiler on high. Coat foil lined baking sheet with cooking spray.

1 ➤ Tomato, fresh, medium, quartered
1 ➤ Pepper, Jalapeno, halved, seeded
½ ➤ Onion, sweet, fresh, cut into wedges
1 ➤ Bell Pepper, any color, sliced

○ Place above ingredients in single layer on a prepared baking sheet.

1 T ➤ Olive Oil
½ t ➤ Oregano, dried
½ t ➤ Chili Powder
¼ t ➤ Cumin, ground
dash ➤ Kosher Salt
dash ➤ Black Pepper, ground

○ Combine all above ingredients except olive oil in small bowl.
Sprinkle seasoning mixture over vegetable mixture; drizzle oil over
vegetable mixture; stir to coat evenly. Move vegetable mixture
towards edges of baking sheet.

2 ➤ Chicken Breasts, 4 oz each, shredded
dash ➤ Kosher Salt
dash ➤ Black Pepper, ground

○ Lay chicken flat in the middle of the baking sheet. Season with salt & pepper.
Cook under broiler for approximately 5 minutes or until the chicken
reaches 165º F and the vegetables are softened and charred.
Move chicken to a bowl, allow to cool, then shred with two forks.

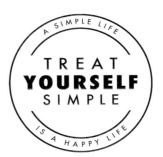

A SIMPLE LIFE
TREAT
YOURSELF
SIMPLE
IS A HAPPY LIFE

4 ➤ Tortilla Shells, 6–8", Flour or Corn
1 ➤ Lime, cut into wedges
¼ C ➤ Salsa
¼ C ➤ Sour Cream
¼ C ➤ Cheese, Mexican, shredded
➤ Cilantro, fresh, chopped

○ Wrap tortillas in paper towels and heat in microwave for 30 seconds; Remove, unwrap, placing 2 tortillas each on two plates.
Divide shredded chicken and roasted vegetables between 4 tortillas. Drizzle with any sauce from the baking sheet. Squeeze lime wedges over tortillas. Divide salsa, sour cream and cheese between 4 tortillas. Serve warm.

NOTES

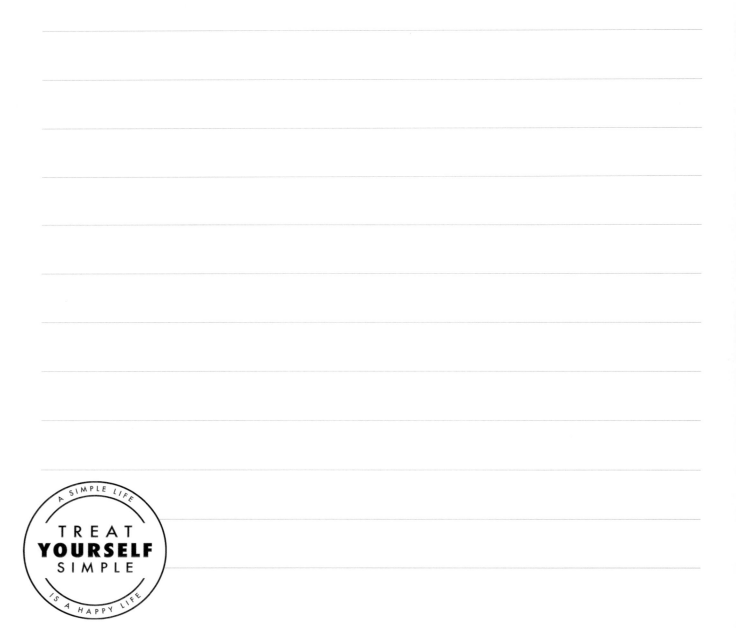

NOTES

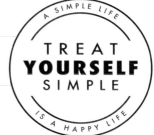

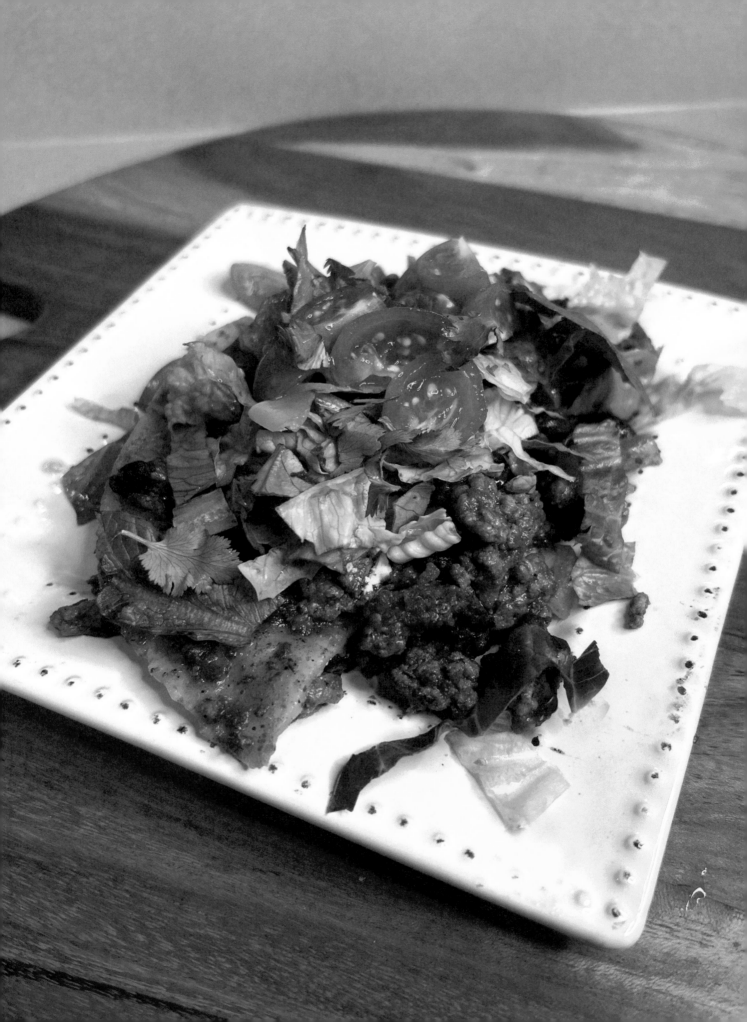

ENCHILADA CASSEROLE 2/1 STOVE/OVEN

Please note: Ground Beef from Taco Stuffed Sweet Potatoes 2/1

Serving Size:	2 servings	Cook time:	30 minutes
Prep time:	25 minutes	Needed:	Skillet, spatula, baking dish, heat-safe spoon

DIRECTIONS

½ lb ‣ Beef, ground, from **Taco Stuffed Sweet Potatoes 2/1**
¼ C ‣ Onion, sweet, chopped

○ In a large skillet, cook beef and onion over medium heat until onion begins to soften and meat is heated through..

½ C ‣ Salsa
¼ can ‣ Beans, black, rinsed and drained, 15 oz can or ½ cup
1 t ‣ Salad Dressing, Italian
½ T ‣ Taco Seasoning
dash ‣ Cumin, ground

○ Stir in the above ingredients to the skillet.

2 ‣ Tortillas Shells, 6–8", Flour or Corn
¼ C ‣ Sour Cream
⅓ C ‣ Cheese, Mexican, shredded

○ Place 1 tortilla in a baking dish coated with cooking spray.
Layer with half of the meat mixture, sour cream, and cheese. Repeat layers.
Cover and bake at 400° F for 25 minutes.

⅓ C ‣ Lettuce, shredded
⅓ C ‣ Tomato, medium, fresh, chopped
to taste ‣ Cilantro, fresh, chopped

○ Uncover. Bake until heated through, 5–10 minutes longer.
Let stand for 5 minutes. Top with lettuce, tomato, and cilantro.
Serve immediately.

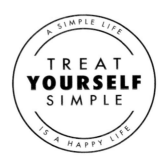

TREAT YOURSELF SIMPLE
A SIMPLE LIFE IS A HAPPY LIFE

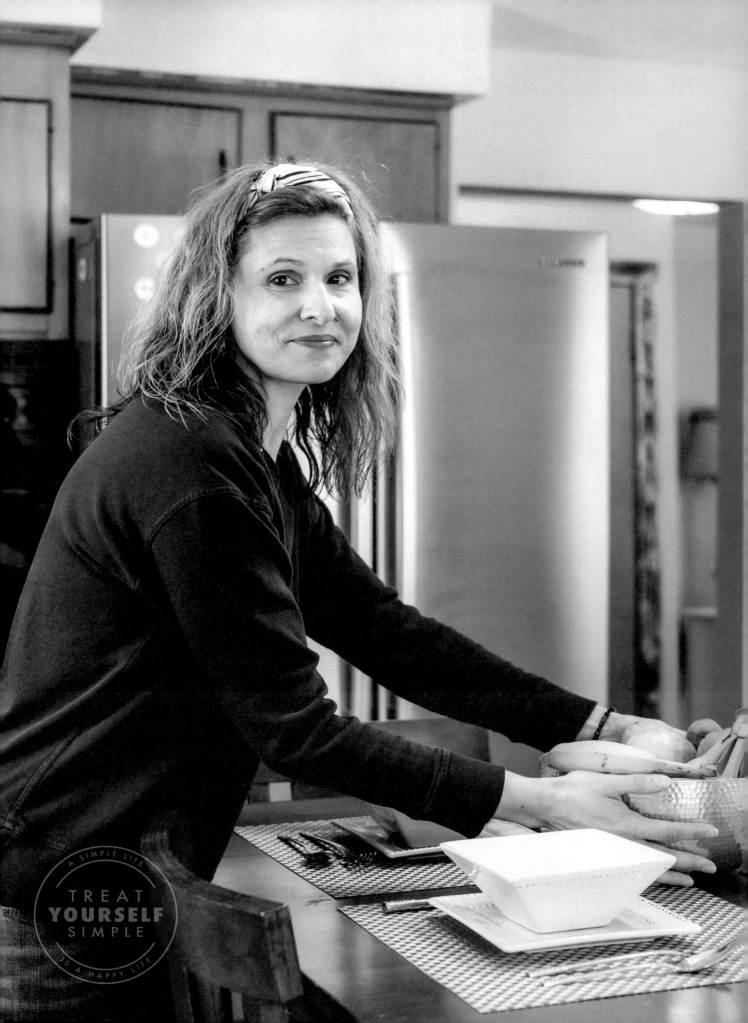

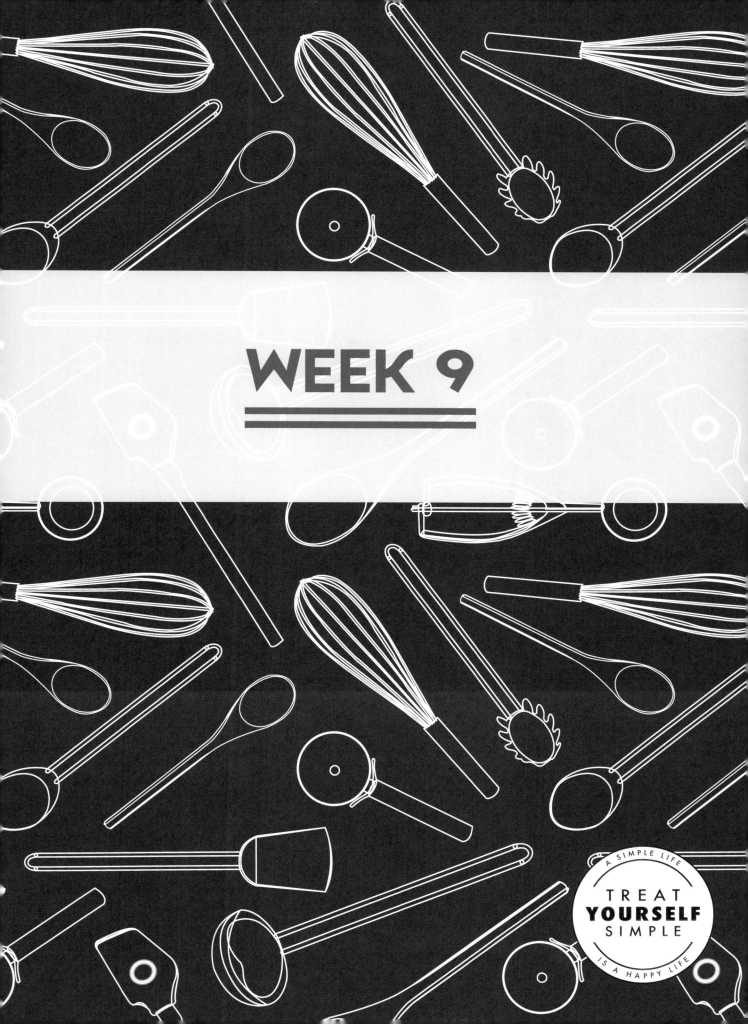

WEEK 9

WEEK 9 MENU PLAN

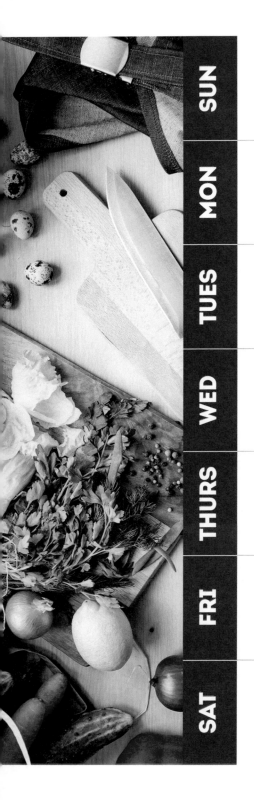

SUN

ROASTED SESAME CHICKEN

Brown Rice
Caesar Salad

MON

ZUCCHINI PIZZA CASSEROLE

Vanilla Yogurt
Cinnamon Sliced Bananas

TUES

PESTO RAVIOLI WITH SPINACH & TOMATOES

Garlic Toast
Fresh Salad

WED

HIGH PLAINS STEAK 2/1

Sweet Potato Discs
Fresh Fruit Bowl

THURS

CORN & POTATO CHOWDER

Coleslaw
Baguette

FRI

BAKED EGGS

Jasmine Rice
Broccoli

SAT

BLACK & BLUE STEAK SALAD 2/1

Cornbread
Coleslaw

WEEK 9 GROCERY LIST

BY MEAL

ROASTED SESAME CHICKEN

2	Chicken Breasts, 4 oz each
¼"	Ginger, fresh, peeled, grated
dash	Kosher Salt
1	Onion, green, fresh, sliced
1 T	Rice Vinegar, unseasoned
1 T	Sesame Oil
½ t	Sesame Seeds, toasted
1 T	Soy Sauce
1 T	Sriracha

ZUCCHINI PIZZA CASSEROLE

dash	Kosher Salt
1	Zucchini, medium, fresh, unpeeled, shredded
1	Egg, large, beaten
2 T + 2 T	Cheese, Cheddar, shredded
¼ C + ¼ C	Cheese, Mozzarella, shredded
2 T + 2 T	Cheese, Parmesan, shredded
½ lb	Beef, ground
2 T	Onion, sweet, fresh, chopped
½ t	Garlic, minced
¼ t	Oregano, dried
1 C	Pasta Sauce
½ t	Seasoning Salt
½ t	Maple Syrup
½ t	Worcestershire Sauce
¼	Bell Pepper, any color, medium, fresh, chopped

PESTO RAVIOLI WITH SPINACH & TOMATOES

2 oz	Spinach, baby, fresh
1 pkg	Cheese Ravioli, fresh or frozen, 8 oz
optional	Cheese, Feta
1 t	Garlic, minced
½ T	Olive Oil
3 T	Pesto
1 pint	Tomatoes, grape or cherry (my fave – Flavorbombs), halved

HIGH PLAINS STEAKS 2/1

1 t	Black Pepper, ground
1 t	Kosher Salt
1 T	Mustard, yellow
2 t	Worcestershire Sauce
4	Sirloin Strip Steaks, 4 oz each, 2 steaks for **Black & Blue Steak Salad 2/1**

CORN & POTATO CHOWDER

¼ C	Cheese, Cheddar, sharp, shredded
1 C	Corn, frozen kernels
¾ C	Bell Pepper, any color, chopped
¼ + ⅛ C	Onions, green, tops only, chopped and divided, about 1 bunch
½ C	Half & Half
⅛ C	Parsley, fresh, chopped
1 C	Potatoes, chopped into bite-sized pieces
dash	Pepper, red, ground
⅓ t	Salt
½ t	Seafood Seasoning (such as Old Bay)
⅓ t	Thyme, dried
¾ C	Water
½ T	Olive Oil

BAKED EGGS

dash	Black Pepper, ground
½ C	Cheese, Colby Jack, shredded
4	Eggs, large
dash	Kosher Salt
1 t	Milk
2 C	Spinach, baby, fresh

BLACK & BLUE STEAK SALAD 2/1

1 T	Vinegar, Balsamic
½ t	Mustard, Dijon
3 T	Olive Oil
¼	Avocado, fresh, sliced
2 C	Spinach, baby, fresh
2 T	Blue Cheese, crumbled
¼ C	Onion, red, sliced
2	Sirloin Strip Steaks, 4 oz. each, from **High Plains Steak 2/1**

WEEK 9 PREP

Mince 3 Garlic cloves ~ Zucchini Pizza Casserole, Pesto Ravioli with Spinach & Tomatoes

Chop 1 Bell Pepper, any color ~ Zucchini Pizza Casserole

Chop ¾ C Bell Pepper, any color ~ Corn & Potato Chowder

Slice ¼ C Red Onion ~ Black & Blue Steak Salad 2/1

Chop ¼ Sweet Onion ~ Zucchini Pizza Casserole

Shred ½ C Cheddar Cheese ~ Zucchini Pizza Casserole, Corn & Potato Chowder

Shred ½ C Mozzarella Cheese ~ Zucchini Pizza Casserole

Shred 4 T Parmesan Cheese ~ Zucchini Pizza Casserole

Shred ½ C Colby Jack Cheese ~ Baked Eggs

WEEK 9 MAKE AHEAD

Make Sauce ~ Roasted Sesame Chicken

Brown Ground Beef with Onion ~ Zucchini Pizza Casserole

Make Dressing ~ Black & Blue Steak Salad 2/1

NOTES

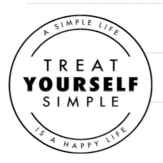

WEEK 9 RECIPES

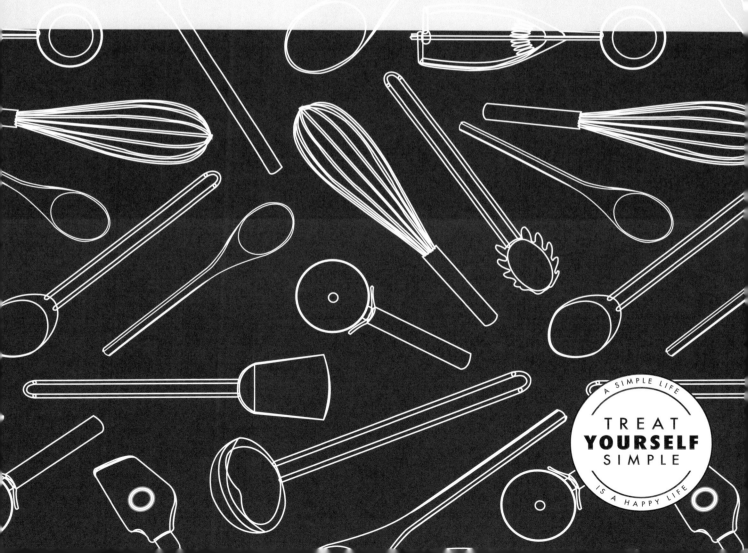

A SIMPLE LIFE

TREAT
YOURSELF
SIMPLE

IS A HAPPY LIFE

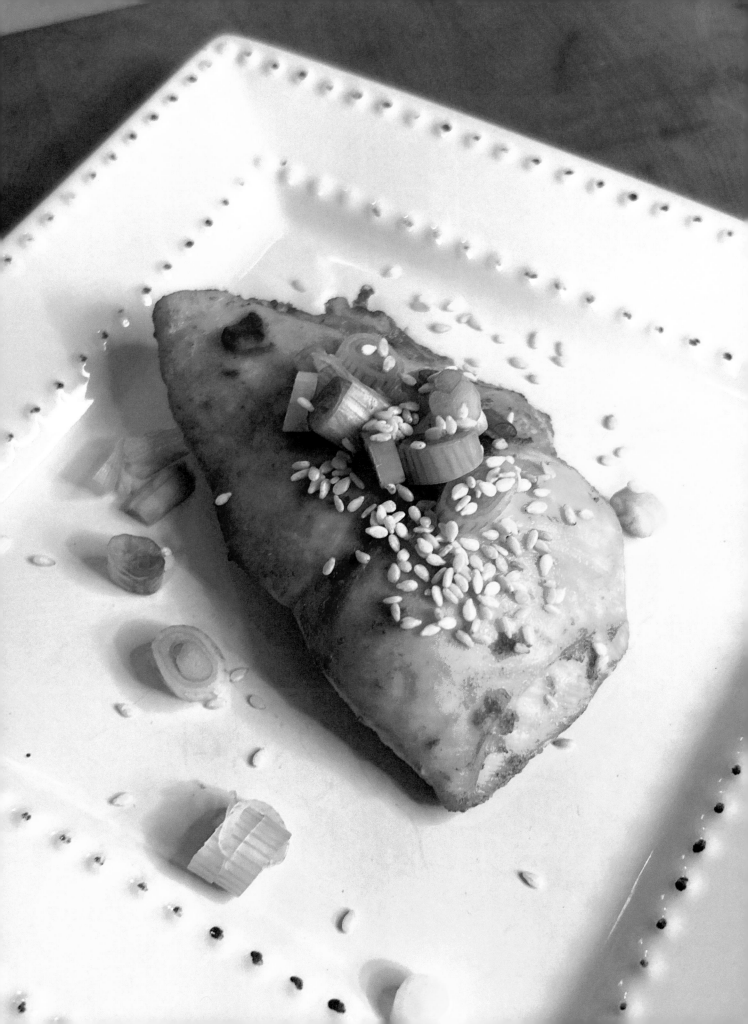

ROASTED SESAME CHICKEN OVEN

Serving Size:	2 servings	Cook time:	20 minutes
Prep time:	15 minutes	Needed:	Baking sheet, small bowl, spatula

DIRECTIONS

2 ➢ Chicken Breasts, 4 oz each
dash ➢ Kosher Salt

○ Preheat oven to 400º F.

○ Place chicken breasts on foil-lined baking sheet with sides. Sprinkle salt over chicken breasts.

¼" ➢ Ginger, fresh, peeled, grated
1 T ➢ Rice Vinegar, unseasoned
1 T ➢ Sesame Oil
1 T ➢ Soy Sauce
1 T ➢ Sriracha

○ In a small bowl, combine the above ingredients. Pour sauce over chicken. Place chicken in oven for 20 minutes.

1 ➢ Onion, green, fresh, sliced
½ t ➢ Sesame Seeds, toasted

○ Place each chicken breast on a plate. Drizzle pan juices over chicken. Top chicken with green onions and sesame seeds. Serve warm.

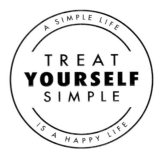

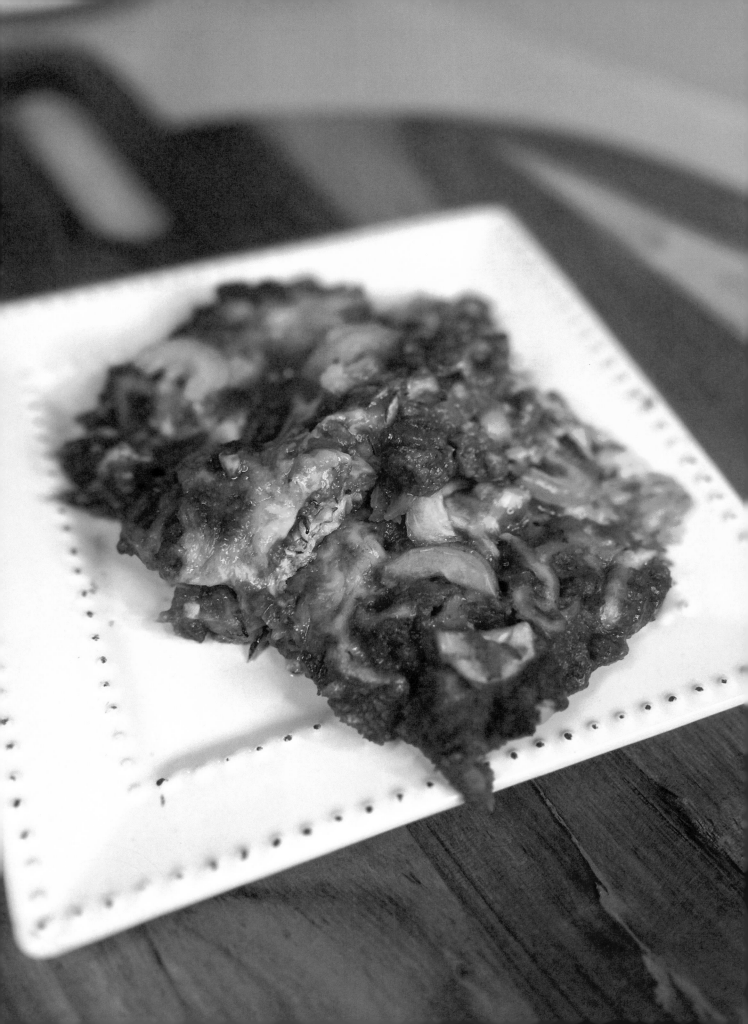

ZUCCHINI PIZZA CASSEROLE OVEN

Serving Size:	2 servings	Cook time:	1 hour
Prep time:	20 minutes	Needed:	Casserole dish, colander, skillet, spatula, spoon

DIRECTIONS

○ Preheat oven to 400º F. Coat a casserole dish with cooking spray. Set aside.

dash ➤ Kosher Salt
1 ➤ Zucchini, medium, fresh, unpeeled, shredded

○ Add, in a colander, the above ingredients. Let stand for 10 minutes; then squeeze out moisture. Add drained zucchini to baking dish set aside.

1 ➤ Egg, large, beaten
2 T ➤ Cheese, Cheddar, shredded
¼ C ➤ Cheese, Mozzarella, shredded
2 T ➤ Cheese, Parmesan, shredded

○ In same baking dish, add above ingredients; combine together to make a crust/bottom for this dish by pressing into the baking dish. Bake for 10 minutes. Remove from heat.

½ lb ➤ Beef, ground

○ **Can make ahead. See Make Ahead Directions.** If not already prepared, add the above ingredients to skillet over medium heat. Brown for 8-10 minutes, breaking meat apart into smaller pieces and combining seasonings, until browned and cooked through.

NOTE: *Mixture can be made ahead and heated when ready to use.*

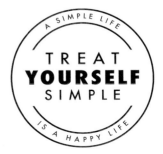

2 T ➤ Onion, sweet, fresh, chopped
½ t ➤ Garlic, minced
¼ t ➤ Oregano, dried
1 C ➤ Pasta Sauce
½ t ➤ Seasoning Salt
½ t ➤ Maple Syrup
½ t ➤ Worcestershire Sauce

○ Add the above ingredients to ground beef in skillet; mix together;
cook for 5–8 minutes until sauce begins to simmer.
Remove from heat; set aside.

¼ ➤ Bell Pepper, any color, medium, fresh, chopped
2 T ➤ Cheese, Cheddar, shredded
¼ C ➤ Cheese, Mozzarella, shredded
2 T ➤ Cheese, Parmesan, shredded

○ Layer on zucchini crust, ground beef mixture, green peppers, and cheeses.
Bake 20 minutes. Serve warm.

NOTES

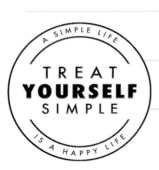

NOTES

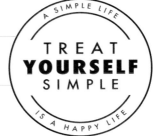

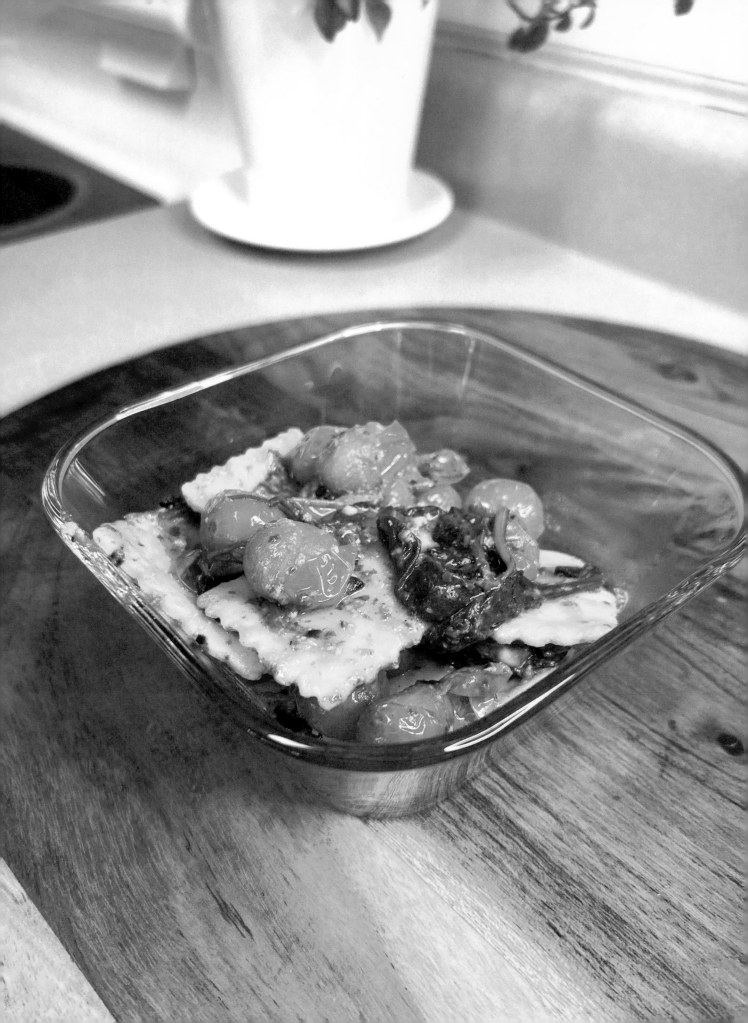

PESTO RAVIOLI WITH SPINACH & TOMATOES   STOVE

Serving Size:	2 servings	Cook time:	25 minutes
Prep time:	15 minutes	Needed:	Medium saucepan, colander, large skillet, heat-safe spoon

DIRECTIONS

1 pkg ➤ Cheese Ravioli. fresh or frozen, 8 oz

○ Bring water to a boil in medium saucepan.
Cook ravioli according to package directions; drain and set aside.

½ T ➤ Olive Oil
1 t ➤ Garlic, minced
1 pint ➤ Tomatoes, grape or cherry (my fave – Flavorbombs), halved

○ Coat skillet with olive oil over medium heat. Add above ingredients;
sauté until tomatoes begin to burst, 3–4 minutes.

2 oz ➤ Spinach, baby, fresh

○ Add above ingredient to skillet and continue to cook, stirring frequently,
until it wilts, 1–2 minutes.

3 T ➤ Pesto

○ Add the cooked ravioli and pesto to the skillet;
stir gently to combine 2–3 minutes. Remove from heat.

optional ➤ Cheese, Feta

○ Divide into two servings in bowls or plates. Sprinkle with above ingredient.
Serve warm.

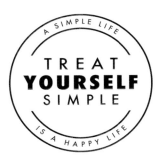

A SIMPLE LIFE
TREAT
YOURSELF
SIMPLE
IS A HAPPY LIFE

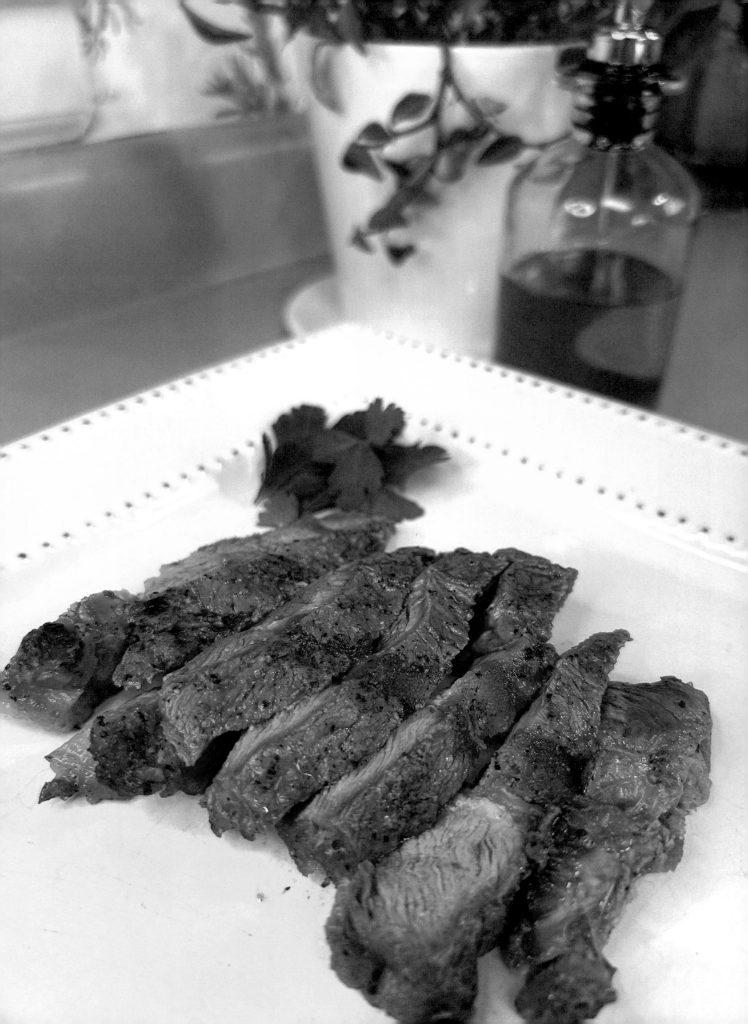

HIGH PLAINS STEAK 2/1 GRILL OR OVEN

Please note: Makes Steak for the Black & Blue Steak Salad 2/1

Serving Size:	2 servings	Cook time:	20 minutes
Prep time:	35 minutes	Needed:	Casserole dish, spatula

DIRECTIONS

○ Preheat oven or grill to 350º F.

1 t ➤ Black Pepper, ground
1 t ➤ Kosher Salt
1 T ➤ Mustard, yellow
2 t ➤ Worcestershire Sauce
4 ➤ Sirloin Strip Steaks, 4 oz. each

○ Combine above ingredients except steak in casserole dish;
rub mixture over both sides of steak; cover and let stand for 30 minutes.

GRILL

○ Place steaks on grill. Grill for 5 -10 minutes, until internal temperature
reaches 145º F. Remove from heat. Let cool for 3–5 minutes.
Place 1 steak on each of two plates. Serve warm.

OVEN

○ Place steaks on foil-lined baking sheet. Bake for 10 minutes,
until internal temperature reaches 145º F. Remove from heat.
Let cool for 3–5 minutes. Place 1 steak each of two plates. Serve warm.

NOTE: *Remove 2 steaks for* **Black & Blue Steak Salad 2/1.**
Set aside, cool, and store in an airtight container. Refrigerate for 7–10 days.

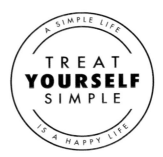

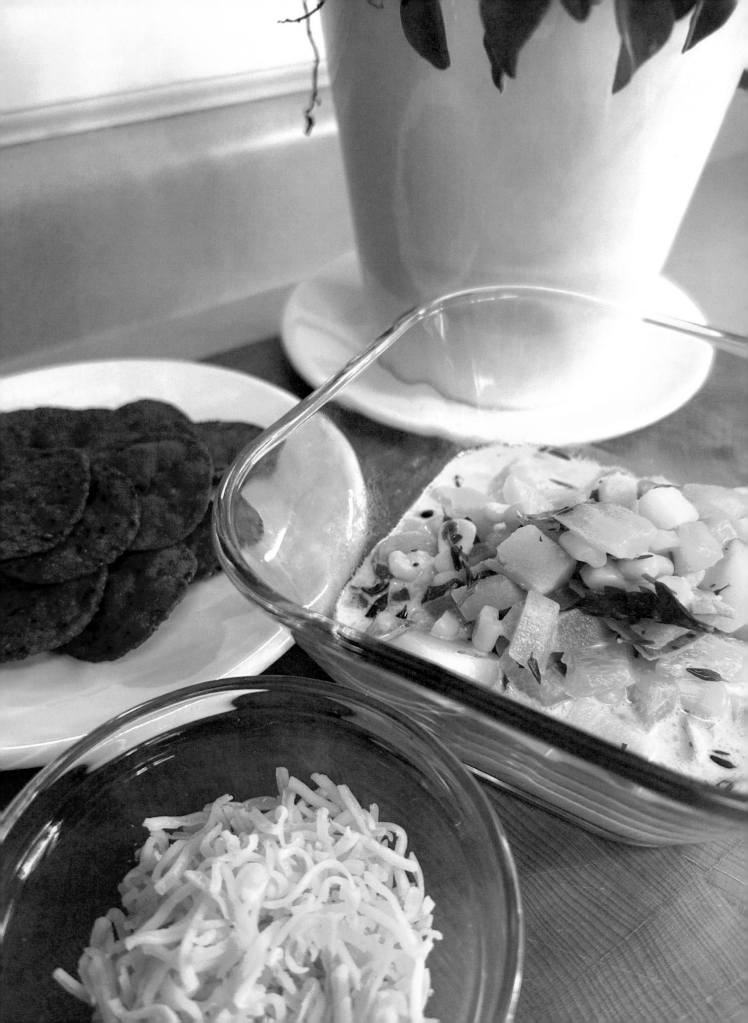

CORN & POTATO CHOWDER STOVE

Serving Size:	2 servings	Cook time:	25 minutes
Prep time:	20 minutes	Needed:	Medium saucepan, heat-safe spoon

DIRECTIONS

½ T ➢ Olive Oil
¾ C ➢ Bell Pepper, any color, chopped
¼ C ➢ Onions, green, tops only, chopped

○ Add above ingredients to medium saucepan over medium heat; sauté 4 minutes or until lightly browned.

1 C ➢ Corn, frozen kernels
¾ C ➢ Water
½ t ➢ Seafood Seasoning (such as Old Bay)
⅓ t ➢ Thyme, dried
dash ➢ Pepper, red, ground
1 C ➢ Potatoes, chopped into bite-sized pieces

○ Increase heat to high. Add above ingredients and bring to a boil.

○ Reduce heat to low, cover, and simmer 10 minutes or until potatoes are tender.

½ C ➢ Half & Half
⅛ C ➢ Parsley, fresh, chopped
⅓ t ➢ Salt

○ Remove from heat. Stir in above ingredients.

○ Divide into two bowls.

¼ C ➢ Cheese, Cheddar, sharp, shredded
⅛ C ➢ Onions, green, tops only, chopped

○ Sprinkle each bowl with cheese and onion. Serve warm.

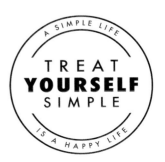

A SIMPLE LIFE
TREAT
YOURSELF
SIMPLE
IS A HAPPY LIFE

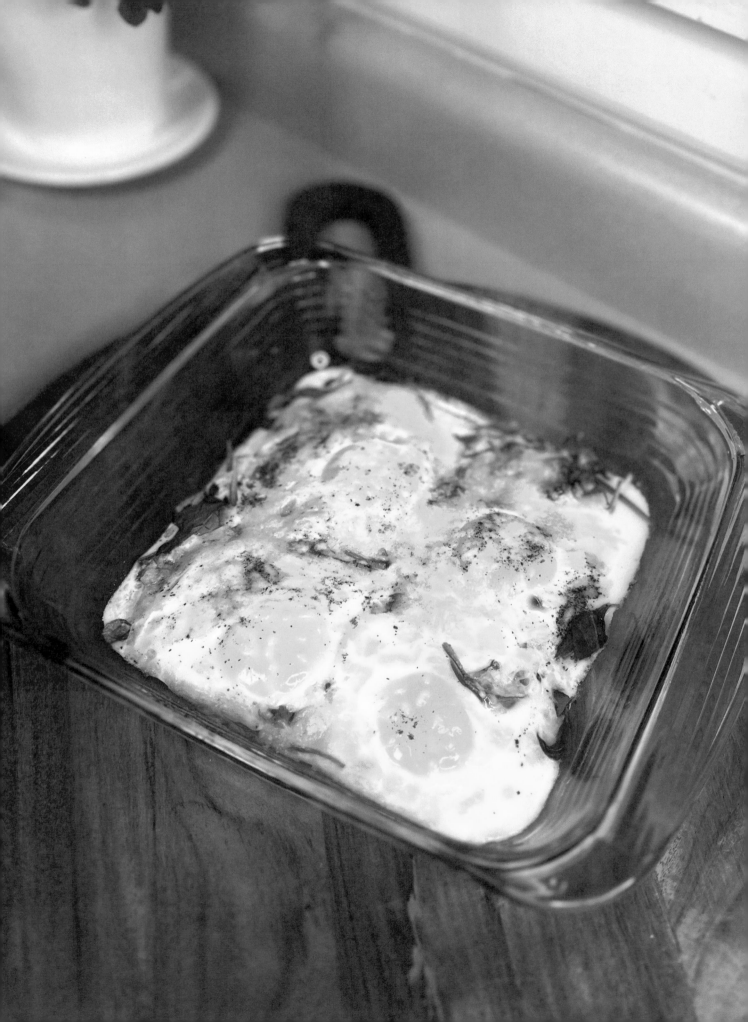

BAKED EGGS OVEN

Serving Size:	2 servings	Cook time:	10 minutes
Prep time:	10 minutes	Needed:	Casserole dish, skillet, heat-safe spoon, spatula

DIRECTIONS

○ Preheat the oven to 350°F. Coat casserole dish with cooking spray. Set aside.

2 C ➢ Spinach, baby, fresh

○ In a large skillet, over high heat, quickly fry the spinach leaves until they are wilted (about 30 seconds). Place the spinach in casserole dish.

4 ➢ Eggs, large

○ Crack the eggs and make sure they cover all the spinach so the cheese sits on the eggs and doesn't leak into the spinach.

½ C ➢ Cheese, Colby Jack, shredded

○ Sprinkle half of the cheese over eggs in casserole dish

1 t ➢ Milk

○ Pour the milk over the cheese in casserole dish

dash ➢ Kosher Salt
dash ➢ Black Pepper, ground

○ Sprinkle with salt & pepper and other half of the cheese.
Bake 8–10 minutes, depending on the oven, until whites are just set and yolks are still runny. Remove from heat. Divide into two servings. Serve warm.

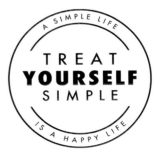

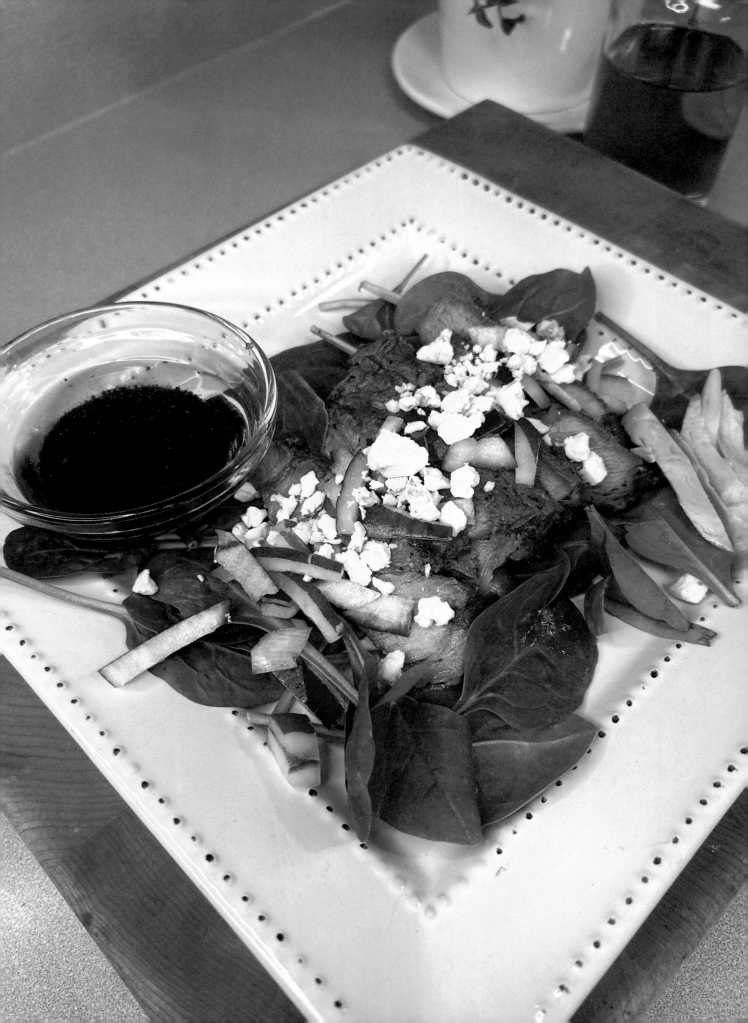

BLACK & BLUE STEAK SALAD 2/1 NO COOK

Please note: Steaks from the High Plains Steak 2/1

Serving Size:	2 servings	**Cook time:**	**No cooking required**
Prep time:	15 minutes	**Needed:**	**Small bowl or measuring cup, spoon**

DIRECTIONS

1 T ➤ Vinegar, Balsamic
½ t ➤ Mustard, Dijon
3 T ➤ Olive Oil

DRESSING

○ **Can make ahead. See Make Ahead Directions.** If not already prepared, add above ingredients in a measuring cup or small bowl; whisk together until well blended; refrigerate until ready to serve.

2 C ➤ Spinach, baby, fresh
¼ C ➤ Onion, red, sliced
 2 ➤ Sirloin Strip Steaks, 4 oz each, from **High Plains Steaks 2/1**, sliced
¼ ➤ Avocado, fresh, sliced
2 T ➤ Blue Cheese, crumbled

○ Split spinach and red onion between two bowls; add the steak; top with avocado, cheese and dressing. Serve immediately.

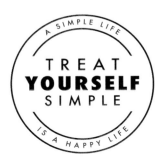

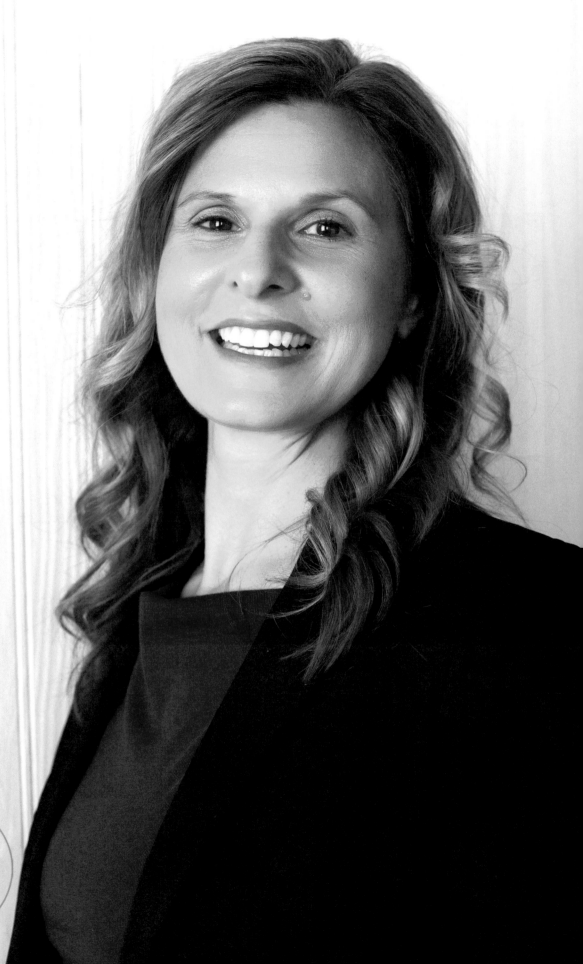

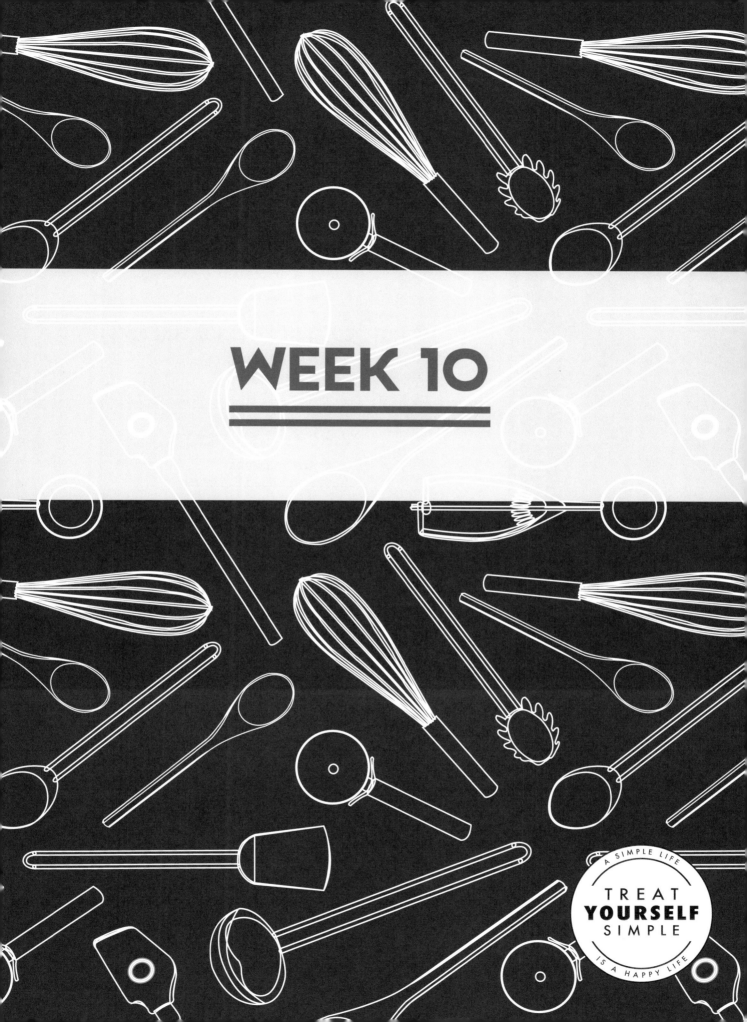

WEEK 10

WEEK 10 MENU PLAN

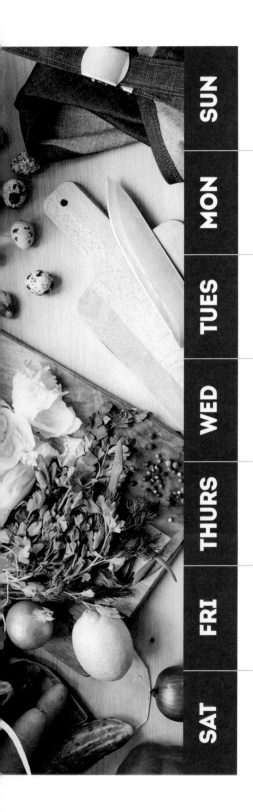

SUN

SLOW COOKER CARNITAS 2/1

Jasmine Rice
Carrots

MON

CHOPPED APPLE QUINOA SALAD

Garlic Toast
Broccoli

TUES

CRUNCHY FISH FILETS

Green Beans
Cinnamon Sliced Bananas

WED

PULLED PORK SLIDERS 2/1

Coleslaw
Orange Slices

THURS

SHRIMP STIR FRY

Jasmine Rice
Fresh Salad

FRI

LOADED VEGETARIAN QUICHE

Coleslaw
Fresh Fruit Bowl

SAT

TACO SOUP

Fresh Salad
Cinnamon Apples

WEEK 10 GROCERY LIST

BY MEAL

SLOW COOKER CARNITAS 2/1

¼ t	Black Pepper, ground
1 t	Cumin, ground
½ t	Garlic, minced
½ t	Kosher Salt
½ T	Olive Oil
¼ C	Orange Juice
½ t	Oregano, dried
1 lb	Pork Tenderloin
¼ C	Onion, sweet, chopped
4	Tortilla Shells, 6–8", Flour or Corn

CHOPPED APPLE QUINOA SALAD

¾ C	Quinoa, cooked, (Success Boil-in-Bag)
½	Apple, large, fresh, chopped
¾ C	Carrot, fresh, matchsticks (purchased at store)
2½ T	Almonds or Walnuts, chopped
1 T	Parsley, fresh, minced
¾ T	Apricot Jam or Preserves
dash	Kosher Salt
2 C	Spinach, baby, fresh

CRUNCHY FISH FILETS

2	Fish Filets, white, 5 oz each
2 T	Breadcrumbs, Panko
½ T	Paprika, ground
dash	Kosher Salt
dash	Black Pepper, ground
1 T	Olive Oil

PULLED PORK SLIDER 2/1

1 t	Olive Oil
½ lb	Slow Cooker Pork from **Pork Carnitas 2/1,** shredded
4	Buns, Slider, split
optional	BBQ Sauce, Cheddar Cheese slices, and/or Pickle slices

SHRIMP STIR FRY

1 T	Olive Oil
½ lb	Broccoli, frozen
½ t	Garlic, minced
½ t	Ginger, fresh, peeled and grated or dash dried ginger
dash	Kosher Salt
1 T	Lemon Juice
½ T	Soy Sauce
12	Shrimp, large, peeled and deveined or 2 C Salad Shrimp

LOADED VEGETARIAN QUICHE

1	Pie Crust, deep dish
1 C	Mushrooms, fresh, sliced
⅓ C	Cheese, Feta, crumbled
1 T	Olive Oil
½ C	Onion, sweet, chopped
½ C	Spinach, fresh or frozen
2 t	Basil, fresh, chopped
2 t	Garlic, minced
2 T	Flour
1	Tomato, medium, fresh, sliced
¼ t	Black Pepper, ground
3	Eggs, large
½ t	Kosher Salt
½ C	Milk
1½ C	Cheese, Mozzarella, shredded

TACO SOUP

½ lb	Beef, ground
⅓ can	Beans, pinto, 15.5 oz can, rinsed and drained
½ C	Corn, frozen
⅓ C	Peas or Edamame, frozen
⅓ can	Beans, black, 15.5 oz can
⅓ can	Tomatoes, diced, 14.5 oz can
⅓ can	Beer, 12 oz can
⅓ can	Tomatoes & Green Chiles, 10 oz can, diced
2 t	Taco Seasoning
2 t	Ranch-style Dressing mix
¼ C	Tortilla Chips, crushed

WEEK 10 PREP

Mince 4 Garlic Cloves ~ Slow Cooker Carnitas 2/1, Shrimp Stir Fry, Loaded Vegetarian Quiche

Slice 1 C Mushrooms ~ Loaded Vegetarian Quiche

Chop ¾ Sweet Onion ~ Slow Cooker Carnitas 2/1, Loaded Vegetarian Quiche

Shred 1½ C Mozzarella Cheese ~ Loaded Vegetarian Quiche

Slice 1 medium Tomato ~ Loaded Vegetarian Quiche

WEEK 10 MAKE AHEAD

Prepare Taco Seasoning ~ Taco Soup

Prepare ¾ C Quinoa (Success Boil-in-Bag) ~ Chopped Apple Quinoa Salad

NOTES

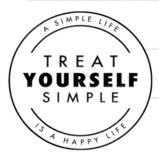

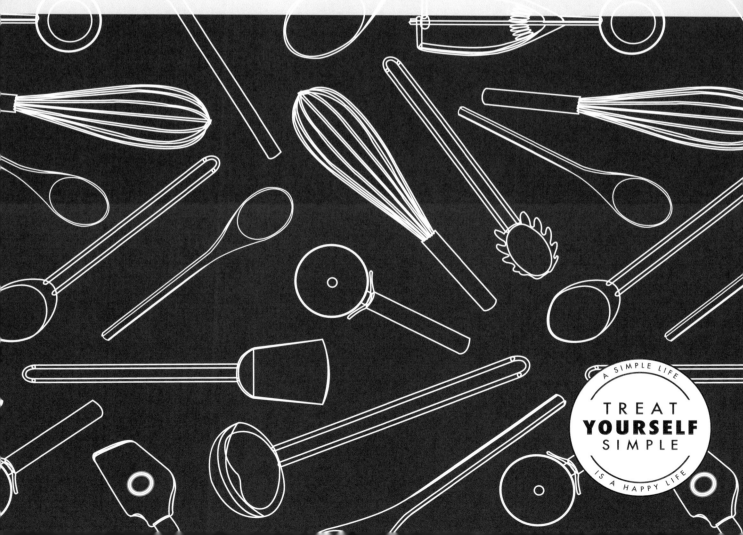

WEEK 10 RECIPES

A SIMPLE LIFE
TREAT
YOURSELF
SIMPLE
IS A HAPPY LIFE

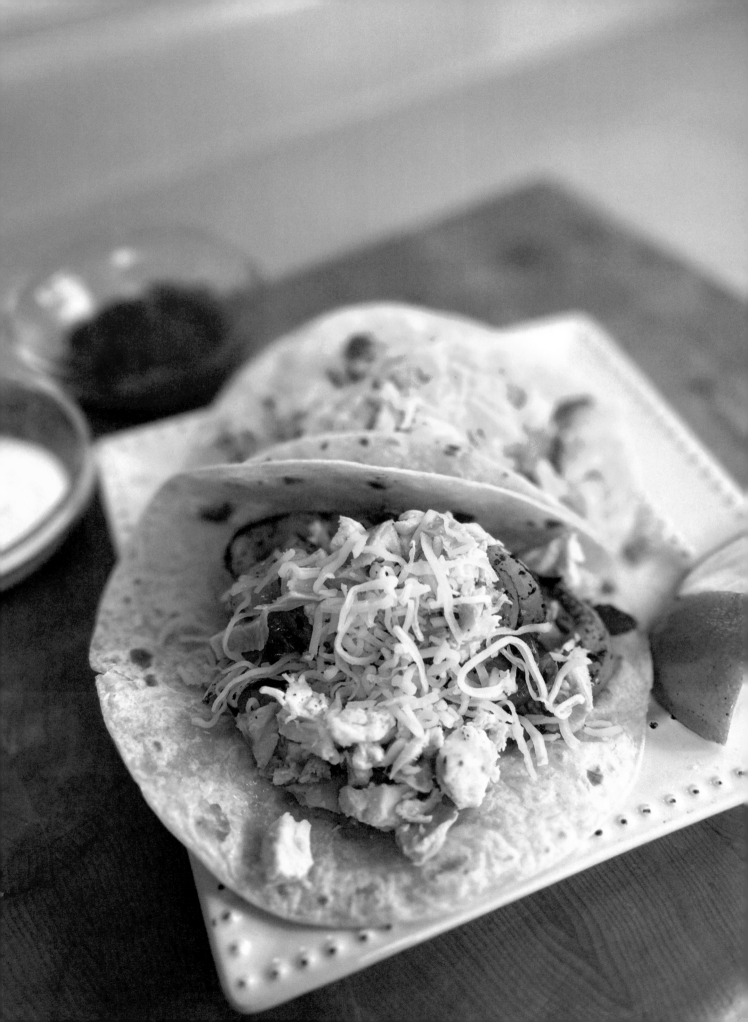

SLOW COOKER CARNITAS 2/1 SLOW COOKER

Please note: Makes Pork for Pulled Pork Sliders 2/1

Serving Size:	2 servings	Cook time:	6 hours
Prep time:	15 minutes	Needed:	Slow cooker, slow cooker liner, plate, medium mixing bowl, tongs

DIRECTIONS

○ In slow cooker, line with slow cooker liner. Turn heat on low.

1 lb ➢ Pork Tenderloin

○ Rinse and dry the pork tenderloin. Place on a plate.

¼ t ➢ Black Pepper, ground
1 t ➢ Cumin, ground
½ t ➢ Kosher Salt
½ T ➢ Olive Oil
½ t ➢ Oregano, dried

○ Combine above ingredients in a medium mixing bowl, then rub all over tenderloin.

½ t ➢ Garlic, minced
¼ C ➢ Onion, sweet, chopped
¼ C ➢ Orange Juice

○ Place pork in a slow cooker, top with above ingredients. Cook on low for10 hours or on high for 6 hours until 145º F is reached.

○ Pork should be tender enough to shred. Remove from slow cooker and let cool slightly. Then shred using two forks.

NOTE: *Remove half of the pork tenderloin for* **Pulled Pork Sliders 2/1.** *Set aside, cool, and store in an airtight container. Refrigerate for 7–10 days.*

4 ➢ Tortilla Shells, 6–8", Flour or Corn

○ Wrap tortillas in paper towels and heat in microwave for 30 seconds; Remove, unwrap, placing 2 tortillas on two plates. Top each shell with one-quarter of the meat.

○ **Top with optional ingredients:** Avocado slices, fresh chopped cilantro, lime juice, shredded Mexican cheese, chopped sweet onions, salsa, sour cream, and/or tomato slices. Seve warm.

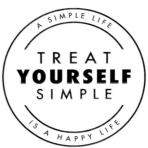

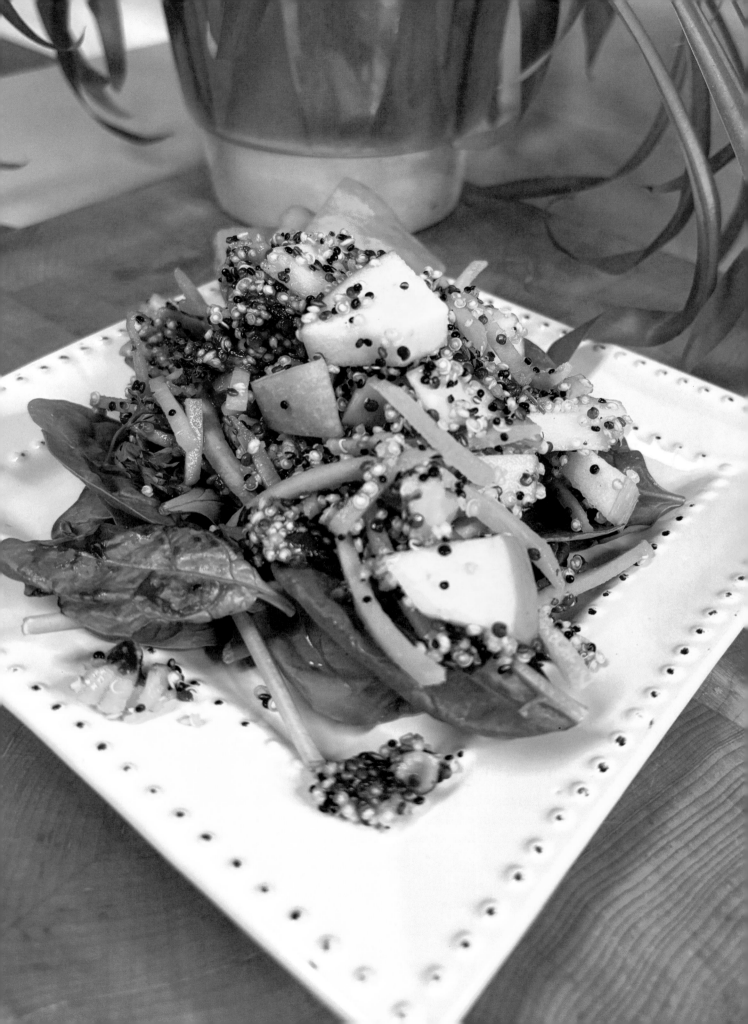

CHOPPED APPLE QUINOA SALAD STOVE

Serving Size:	2 servings	Cook time:	20 minutes
Prep time:	5 minutes	Needed:	Medium saucepan, medium bowl, heat-safe spoon

DIRECTIONS

¾ C ➤ Quinoa, cooked, (Success Boil-in-Bag)

○ Follow package instructions. Remove from heat and cool completely. Place in medium bowl.

½ ➤ Apple, large, fresh, chopped
¾ C ➤ Carrot, fresh, matchsticks (purchased at store)
2 ½ T ➤ Almonds or Walnuts, chopped
1 T ➤ Parsley, fresh, minced
¾ T ➤ Apricot Jam or Preserves
dash ➤ Kosher Salt

○ Add above ingredients to quinoa in bowl; toss until well combined.

2 C ➤ Spinach, baby, fresh

○ Divide spinach on two plates. Divide the apple/quinoa mixture on the spinach on each plate. Enjoy immediately.

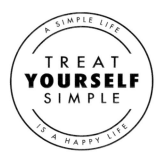

A SIMPLE LIFE
TREAT
YOURSELF
SIMPLE
IS A HAPPY LIFE

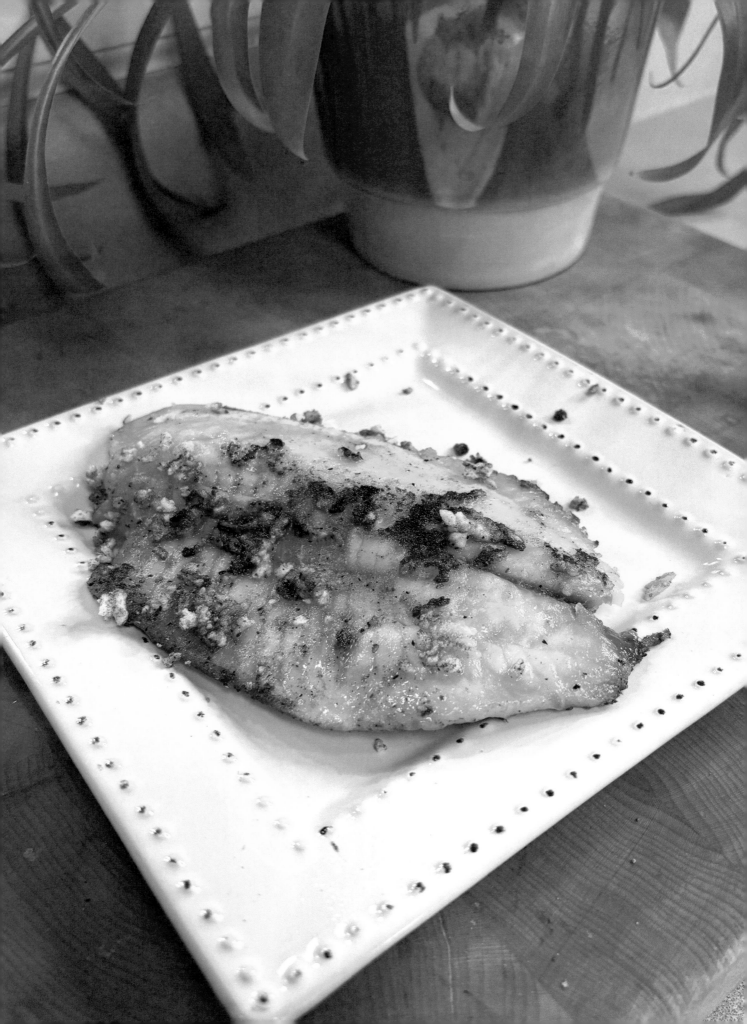

CRUNCHY FISH FILETS OVEN

Serving Size:	2 servings	Cook time:	8 minutes
Prep time:	5 minutes	Needed:	Medium bowl, large skillet, spatula

DIRECTIONS

2 ➤ Fish Filets, white, 5 oz each
2 T ➤ Breadcrumbs, Panko
½ T ➤ Paprika, ground
dash ➤ Kosher Salt
dash ➤ Black Pepper, ground

○ Combine above ingredients, except fish in a medium mixing bowl. Dredge filets in mixture; lightly coat with cooking spray.

1 T ➤ Olive Oil

○ Coat skillet with olive oil over medium heat. Place coated filets in skillet; cook 3–4 minutes per side until fish begins to flake and internal temperature reaches 145° F. Serve warm.

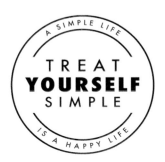

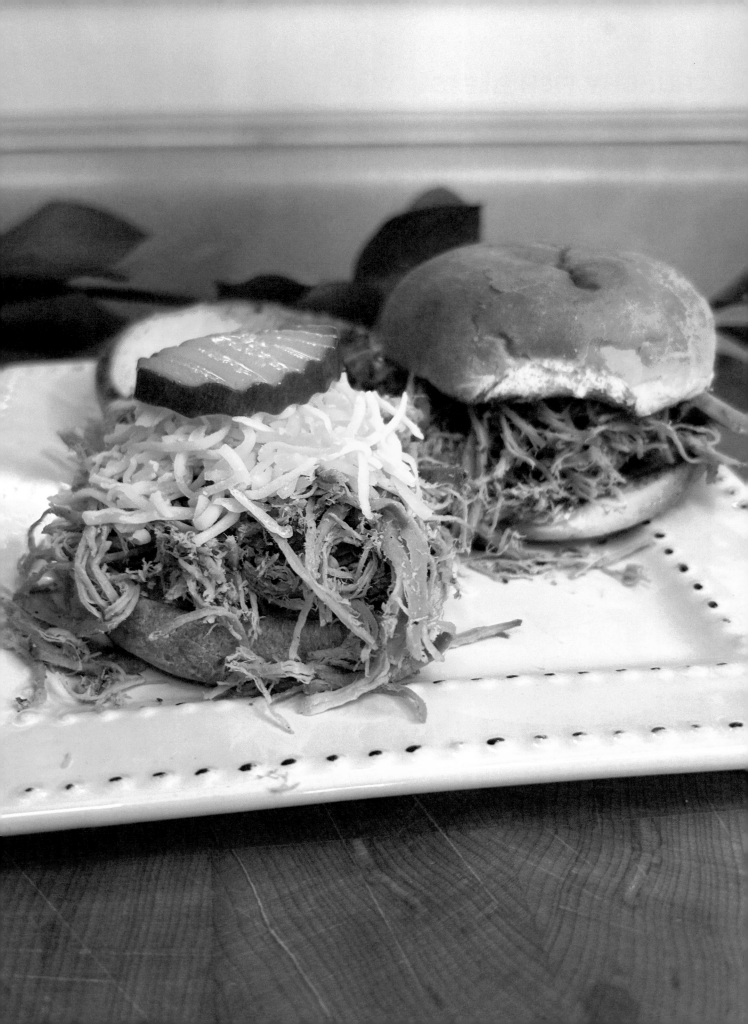

PULLED PORK SLIDERS 2/1 STOVE

Please note: Pork was prepared from Slow Cooker Carnitas 2/1

Serving Size:	2 servings	Cook time:	10 minutes
Prep time:	5 minutes	Needed:	Large skillet, plate, fork, heat-safe spoon

DIRECTIONS

1 t ➤ Olive Oil

○ In a large skillet over medium heat, coat with olive oil.

½ lb ➤ Pork Tenderloin, shredded, from **Slow Cooker Carnitas 2/1**

○ Add shredded pork from carnitas to skillet; stirring occasionally until heated through. Remove from pan, place on plate to put in microwave to keep warm. Wipe out pan with paper towel.

4 ➤ Buns, Slider, split

○ Heat wiped out pan over medium heat. Place buns flat side down, heat until golden browned and warmed. Remove from heat.

optional ➤ BBQ Sauce, Cheddar Cheese slices, and/or Pickle slices.

○ Top each bun with half of the meat. Add optional toppings. Serve warm.

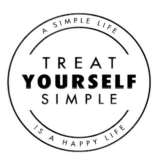

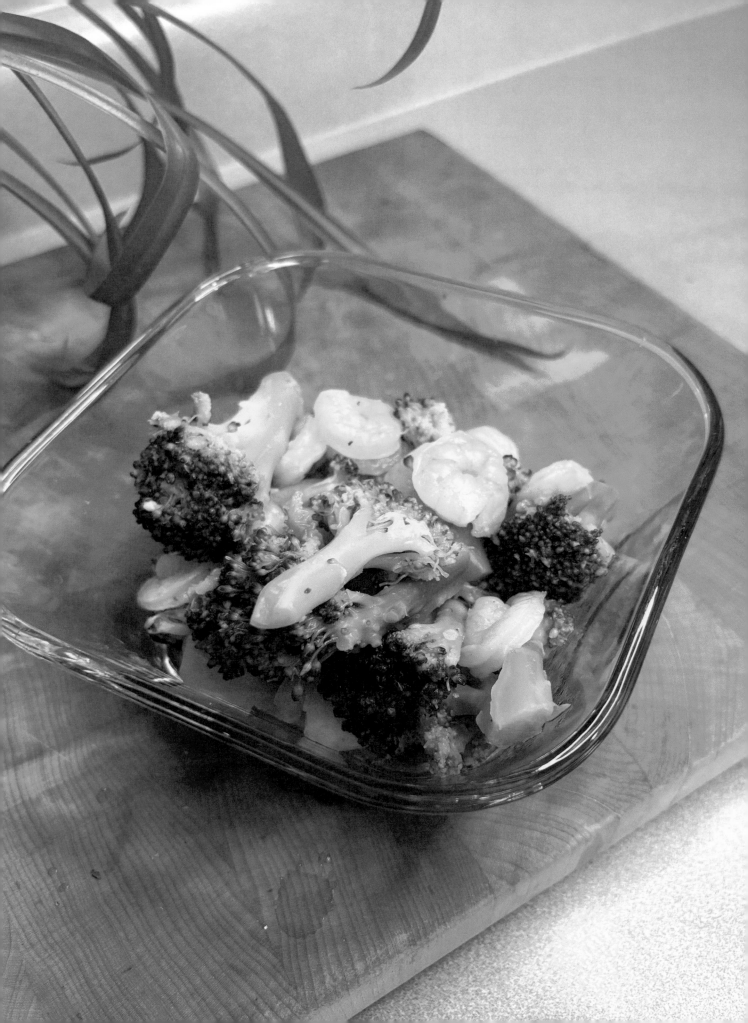

SHRIMP STIR FRY STOVE

Serving Size:	2 servings	Cook time:	10 minutes
Prep time:	10 minutes	Needed:	Large skillet, heat-safe spoon

DIRECTIONS

1 T ➤ Olive Oil
½ lb ➤ Broccoli, frozen
½ t ➤ Garlic, minced
½ t ➤ Ginger, fresh, peeled and grated or dash of dried ginger
dash ➤ Kosher Salt

○ Coat skillet with olive oil over medium heat. Add above ingredients. Stir frequently and cook until broccoli is tender-crisp.

1 T ➤ Lemon Juice
½ T ➤ Soy Sauce

○ Add above ingredients to skillet. Stir until well combined.

12 ➤ Shrimp, large, peeled and deveined or 2 C Salad Shrimp

○ Add shrimp. Stir to combine. Cover and cook for 3 minutes. Divide between two plates or bowls. Serve warm.

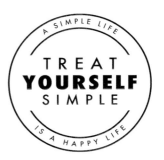

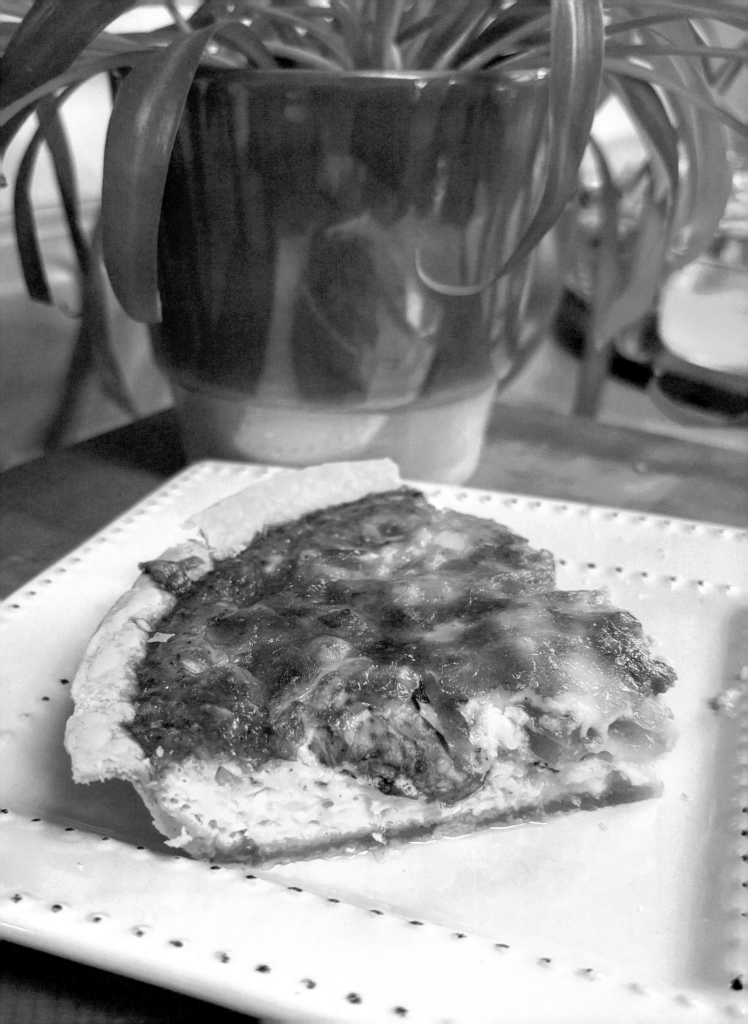

LOADED VEGETAR!AN QUICHE   OVEN

Serving Size:	2 servings	Cook time:	55 minutes
Prep time:	20 minutes	Needed:	Casserole dish, large skillet, measuring cup or small bowl, whisk, heat-safe spoon

DIRECTIONS

○ Preheat oven to 400° F. Coat casserole dish with cooking spray. Set aside.

1 ➤ Pie Crust, deep dish

○ Spread pie crust into casserole dish or leave in pie pan in which the pie crust came. Bake until pie crust is firm; check after 10 minutes, bake 5 more minutes if needed. Remove from heat. Set aside.

1 C ➤ Mushrooms, fresh, sliced
⅓ C ➤ Cheese, Feta, crumbled
1 T ➤ Olive Oil
½ C ➤ Onion, sweet, chopped
½ C ➤ Spinach, fresh or frozen

○ Reduce oven to 350° F. Coat large skillet with olive oil over medium heat. Add the above ingredients; cook for 5–7 minutes, stirring occasionally until vegetables are soft. Remove from skillet. Set aside.

2 t ➤ Basil, fresh, chopped
2 t ➤ Garlic, minced
2 T ➤ Flour
1 ➤ Tomato, fresh, medium, sliced

○ Sprinkle tomato slices with above ingredients; cook in same skillet for 1 minute per side.

¼ t ➤ Black Pepper, ground
3 ➤ Eggs, large
½ t ➤ Kosher Salt
½ C ➤ Milk

○ Combine the above ingredients in a measuring cup or small bowl; whisk together. Set aside.

1½ C ➤ Cheese, Mozzarella, shredded

○ Spread 1 cup of cheese on prepared crust; layer vegetable mixture, prepared tomato slices, egg mixture and remaining ½ cup cheese. Bake for 40–45 minutes until a knife inserted near the center comes out clean. Cool 5 minutes before serving. Serve warm.

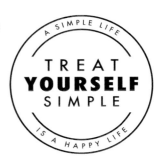

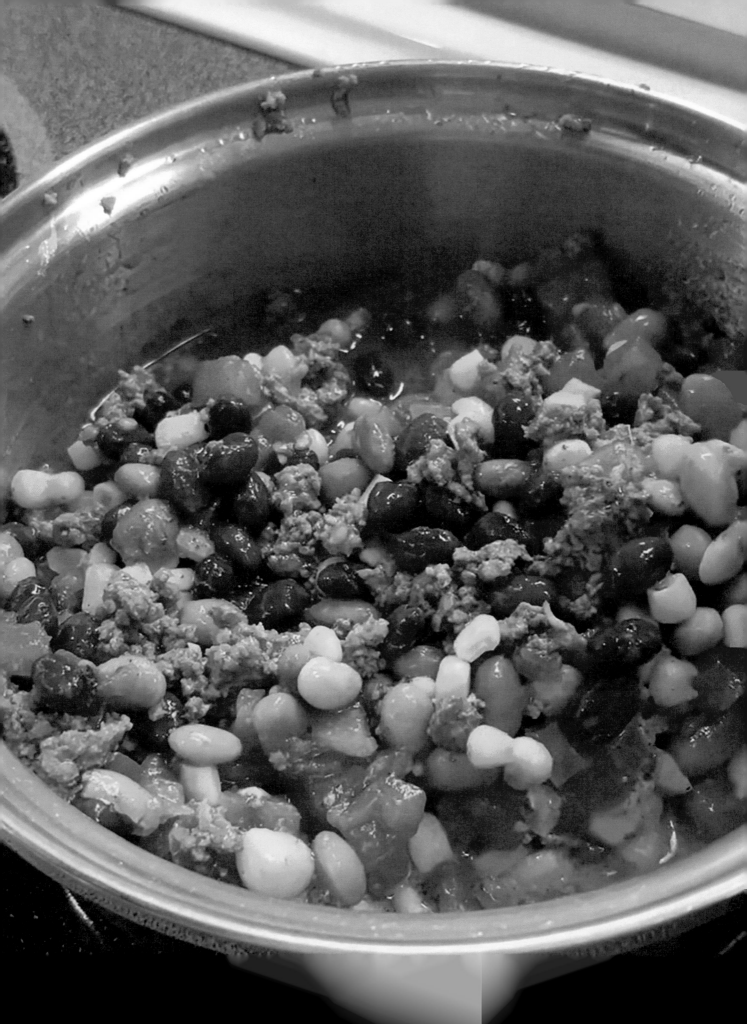

TACO SOUP STOVE

Serving Size:	2 servings	Cook time:	40 minutes
Prep time:	15 minutes	Needed:	Medium saucepan, heat-safe spoon

DIRECTIONS

½ lb ➤ Beef, ground

○ Brown beef in a medium saucepan, stirring until crumbled and is no longer pink; drain if needed.

⅓ can ➤ Beans, pinto, 15.5 oz can, rinsed and drained
½ C ➤ Corn, frozen
⅓ C ➤ Peas or Edamame, frozen
⅓ can ➤ Beans, black, 15.5 oz can
⅓ can ➤ Tomatoes, diced, 14.5 oz can
⅓ can ➤ Beer, 12 oz can
⅓ can ➤ Tomatoes & Green Chiles, 10 oz can, diced
2 t ➤ Taco Seasoning
2 t ➤ Ranch-style Dressing mix

○ Add above ingredients to pan; stir to combine; bring to a boil. Reduce heat; simmer 30 minutes.

¼ C ➤ Tortilla Chips, crushed

○ Ladle soup into bowls and top with tortilla chips. Serve warm.

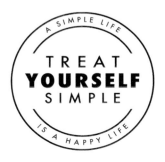

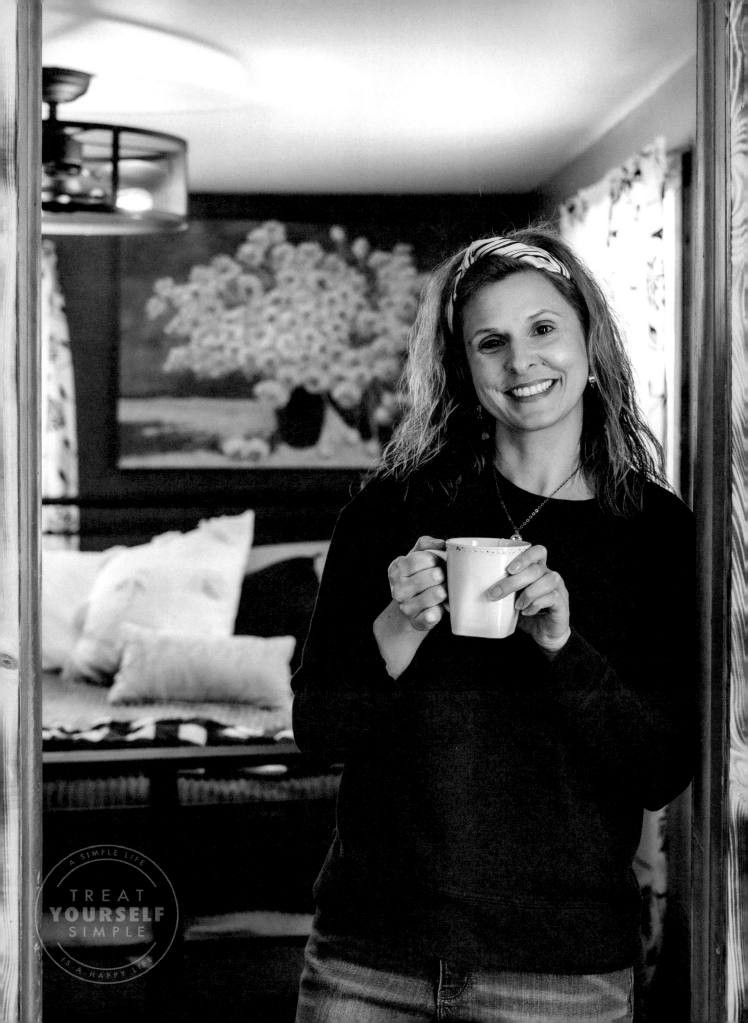

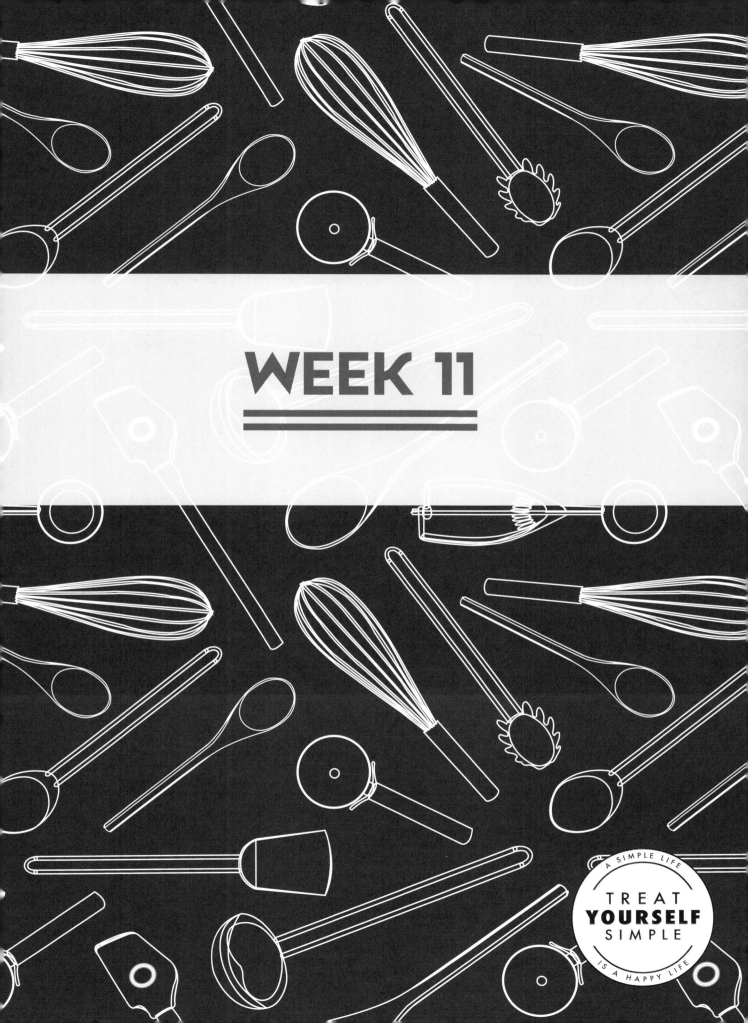

WEEK 11

WEEK 11 MENU PLAN

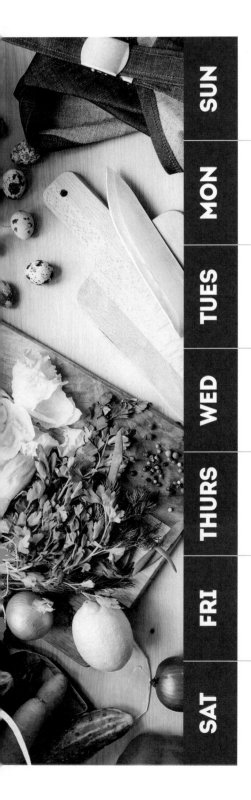

SUN

SPICED CHICKEN WITH APPLES
Jasmine Rice
Green Beans (I prefer french-style)

MON

PASTA WITH PUMPKIN & SAUSAGE 2/1
Orange Slices
Cucumber Slices

TUES

AUTUMN MEXICAN CASSEROLE
Fresh Salad
Fresh Fruit Bowl

WED

BEEF & VEGETABLE STIR FRY
Jasmine Rice
Orange Slices

THURS

VEGGIE FRITTATA WITH SAUSAGE 2/1
Garlic Toast
Fresh Salad

FRI

ASIAN SALMON
Butternut Squash
Fresh Fruit Bowl

SAT

ONE PAN HARVEST PASTA
Fresh Salad
Cinnamon or Spice Apples

WEEK 11 GROCERY LIST

SPICED CHICKEN WITH APPLES

⅛ t	Nutmeg, ground
⅛ t	Cinnamon, ground
⅛ t	Ginger, ground
dash	Cumin, ground
dash	Kosher Salt
dash	Black Pepper, ground
1 T + ½ T	Olive Oil
2	Chicken Breasts, 4 oz each
1	Apple, cut into wedges
1	Onion, red, sliced
2 T	Lemon Juice
¼ C	Chicken Broth
½ T	Maple Syrup
1½ t	Garlic, minced

PASTA WITH PUMPKIN & SAUSAGE 2/1

1 C	Pasta, penne
1 T	Olive Oil
1 lb	Italian Sausage, ground, ½ lb for **Veggie Frittata with Sausage 2/1**
½ T	Olive Oil
1 T	Garlic, minced
½ C	Onion, sweet, chopped
1	Bay leaf
¼ t	Sage, dried
1 C	Stock, Chicken
½ C	Cheese, Mozzarella, shredded
¼ C	Onion, green, sliced
½ C	Pumpkin, canned
¼ C	Cream, heavy
dash	Cinnamon, ground
¼ t	Nutmeg, ground
dash	Kosher Salt
dash	Black Pepper, ground

AUTUMN MEXICAN CASSEROLE

1	Bell Pepper, any color, chopped
¼	Pepper, Jalapeno, diced
2 T	Onion, red, chopped
⅓ C	Corn, fresh or frozen
¼ t	Chili Powder
½ t	Cumin, ground
dash	Kosher Salt
¾ C	Cheese, Mexican, shredded
4	Tortillas, Corn, cut into thin strips
½	Refried Beans, canned (mix with a little bit of water to make them easier to spread)
⅓ C	Enchilada Sauce
	Cilantro, fresh
	Avocado slices
	Sour Cream

BEEF & VEGETABLE STIR FRY

1 T	Olive Oil
1 pkg	Vegetables, mixed, frozen, 10 oz or use 2 C whatever fresh veggies you like
1 t	Flour
½ C	Stir Fry Sauce
1 C	Beef, roast, cut into bite-sized pieces

VEGGIE FRITTATA WITH SAUSAGE 2/1

½ lb	Sausage, ground, from **Pasta with Pumpkin & Sausage 2/1**
¾ C	Spinach, baby, fresh
¼ C	Bell Pepper, any color, chopped
¾ C	Mushrooms, any type, fresh, sliced
¼ C	Onion, sweet, fresh, chopped
4	Eggs, large, beaten
½ C	Milk, any type
2 t	Kosher Salt
dash	Black Pepper, ground
½ C	Cheese, Cheddar, shredded

BY MEAL

ASIAN SALMON

2	Salmon Filets, 4–6 oz
1 t	Ginger, fresh, peeled and grated or ¼ t ground Ginger
1 t	Garlic, minced
1 T	Soy Sauce
2 T	Worcestershire Sauce
2 T	Sriracha Sauce
½ t	Sesame Seeds, toasted
1	Onion, green, chopped

ONE PAN HARVEST PASTA

1 T	Olive Oil
1 C	Eggplant, small, fresh, cut into bite-sized pieces
¼	Zucchini, medium, fresh, chopped
1	Tomato, small, fresh, medium, chopped
1 T	Onion, red, fresh, chopped
½ t	Garlic, minced
¼ can	Beans, cannellini, 15.5 oz can, rinsed and drained
½ C	Broth, Chicken
½ C	Pasta, elbow macaroni
dash	Kosher Salt
dash	Black Pepper, ground
optional	Basil, fresh, chopped
optional	Cheese, Parmesan, shredded

WEEK 11 PREP

Mince 12 Garlic cloves ~ Spiced Chicken with Apples, Asian Salmon, Pasta with Pumpkin & Sausage 2/1, One Pan Harvest Pasta

Chop 1 Bell Pepper, any color ~ Autumn Mexican Casserole

Slice ¼ C Bell Pepper, any color ~ Veggie Frittata with Sausage

Cut 1 C Eggplant into bite-sized pieces ~ One-Pan Harvest Pasta

Chop 3 T Red Onion ~ Autumn Mexican Casserole, One-Pan Harvest Pasta

Slice 1 Red Onion ~ Spiced Chicken with Apples

Chop ¾ Sweet Onion ~ Pasta with Pumpkin & Sausage 2/1, Veggie Frittata with Sausage 2/1

Chop 1 C Tomato ~ One-Pan Harvest Pasta

Chop ¼ Zucchini ~ One-Pan Harvest Pasta

Slice ¾ C Mushrooms, any type ~ Veggie Frittata with Sausage 2/1

Shred ½ C Cheddar Cheese ~ Veggie Frittata with Sausage 2/1

Shred ¾ C Mexican Cheese ~ Autumn Mexican Casserole

Shred ½ C Mozzarella Cheese ~ Pasta with Pumpkin & Sausage 2/1

Cut Beef Roast into bite-sized pieces ~ Beef & Vegetable Stir Fry

WEEK 11 MAKE AHEAD

Prepare Marinade ~ Asian Salmon

Brown Italian Sausage ~ Pasta with Pumpkin & Sausage 2/1, Veggie Frittata with Sausage 2/1

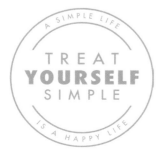

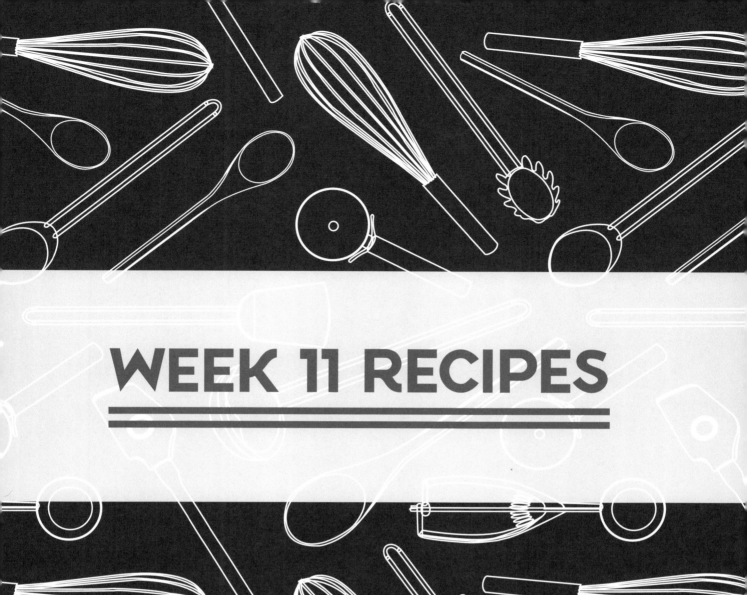

WEEK 11 RECIPES

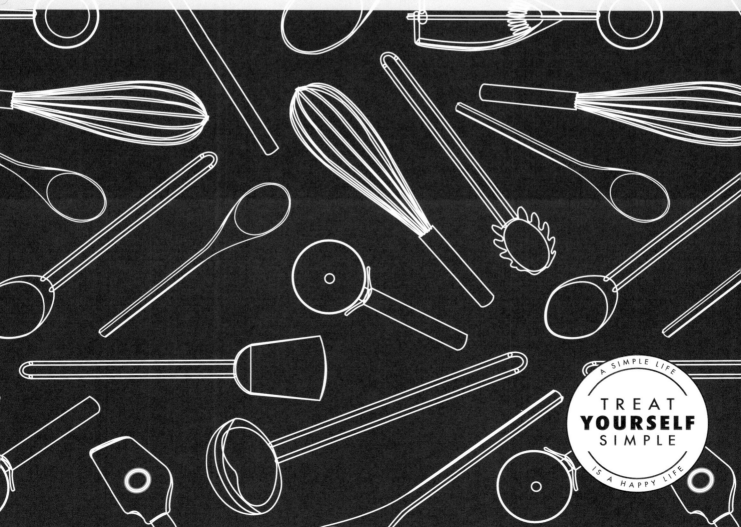

TREAT
YOURSELF
SIMPLE

A SIMPLE LIFE
IS A HAPPY LIFE

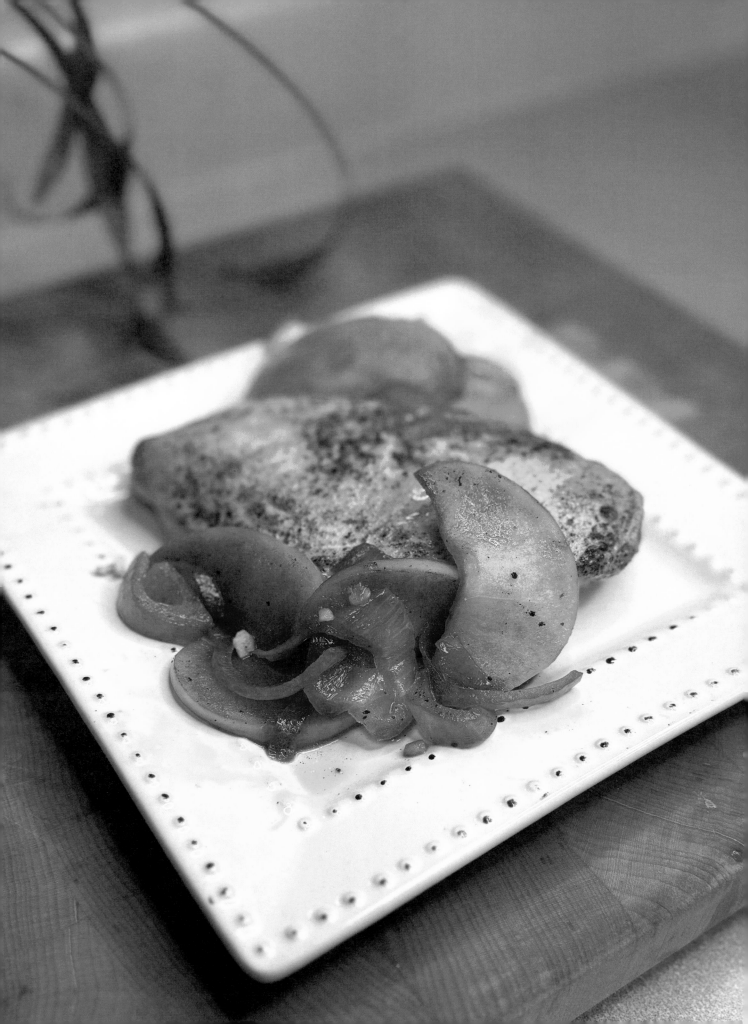

SPICED CHICKEN WITH APPLES STOVE

Serving Size:	2 servings	Cook time:	25 minutes
Prep time:	15 minutes	Needed:	Skillet, small bowl, spatula

DIRECTIONS

⅛ t ➤ Nutmeg, ground
⅛ t ➤ Cinnamon, ground
⅛ t ➤ Ginger, ground
dash ➤ Cumin, ground
dash ➤ Kosher Salt
dash ➤ Black Pepper, ground

○ Combine ingredients into small bowl. Set aside.

1 T ➤ Olive Oil
2 ➤ Chicken Breasts, 4 oz each

○ Coat skillet with olive oil over medium-high heat. Sprinkle chicken with seasoning mix. Cook 3–4 minutes per side until browned. Remove from heat, slice chicken. Set aside.

½ T ➤ Olive Oil
1 ➤ Apple, cut into wedges
1 ➤ Onion, red, sliced

○ Coat same skillet with olive oil over medium heat. Add the above ingredients. Cook until softened and lightly browned, about 4 minutes, stirring occasionally.

2 T ➤ Lemon Juice
¼ C ➤ Chicken Broth
½ T ➤ Maple Syrup
1½ t ➤ Garlic, minced

○ Add above ingredients to skillet. Bring to a boil, then reduce the heat to maintain a simmer.

○ Add chicken on top of apple mixture in skillet. Cover and cook until the chicken is cooked through and sauce is slightly reduced, about 6 minutes.

○ Place one chicken breast on each of two plates. Spoon apple mixture over the chicken breast. Serve warm.

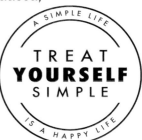

A SIMPLE LIFE
TREAT
YOURSELF
SIMPLE
IS A HAPPY LIFE

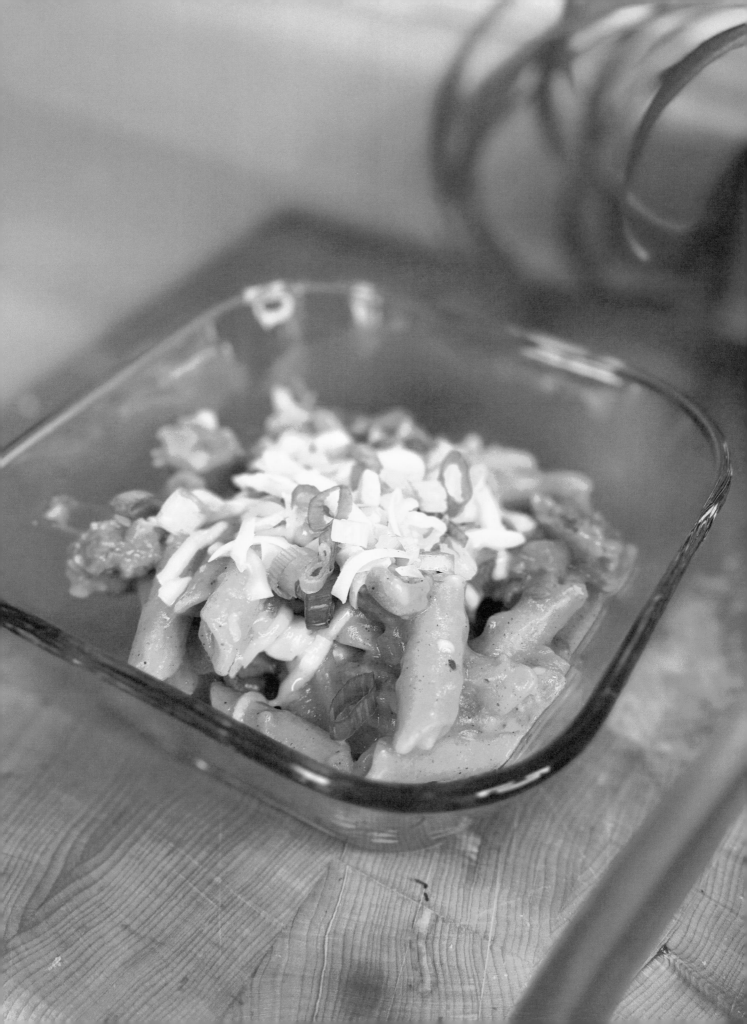

PASTA WITH PUMPKIN & SAUSAGE 2/1 STOVE

Please note: Makes Italian Sausage for Veggie Frittata with Sausage 2/1

Serving Size:	2 servings	**Cook time:**	25 minutes
Prep time:	10 minutes	**Needed:**	Skillet, medium saucepan, heat-safe spoon

DIRECTIONS

1 C ➤ Pasta, penne

○ Cook pasta as directed on package; drain. Set aside.

1 T ➤ Olive Oil
1 lb ➤ Italian Sausage, ground

○ **Can make ahead. See Make Ahead Directions.** If not already prepared, coat skillet with olive oil over medium heat. Add sausage; break meat apart into small pieces, stirring occasionally until fully browned. Transfer sausage to paper towel-lined plate. Drain fat from skillet and return half of the sausage to pan.

NOTE: *Remove half of the Italian sausage for* **Veggie Frittata with Sausage 2/1.** *Set aside, cool, and store in an airtight container. Refrigerate for 7–10 days.*

½ T ➤ Olive Oil
1 T ➤ Garlic, minced
½ C ➤ Onion, sweet, chopped

○ Add above ingredients to skillet. Saute 3–5 minutes until the onion is tender.

1 ➤ Bay leaf
¼ t ➤ Sage, dried
1 C ➤ Stock, Chicken
½ C ➤ Pumpkin, canned
¼ C ➤ Cream, heavy

○ Add above ingredients to the skillet. Return sausage to the pan, reduce heat, stir to combine.

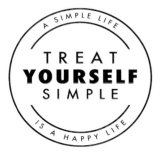

dash ➤ Cinnamon, ground
¼ t ➤ Nutmeg, ground
dash ➤ Kosher Salt
dash ➤ Black Pepper, ground

○ Add above ingredients.
Simmer mixture 5–10 minutes to thicken sauce.

½ C ➤ Cheese, Mozzarella, shredded
¼ C ➤ Onion, green, sliced

○ Remove the bay leaf from sauce. Add cooked pasta to the skillet,
stirring to combine; cook for 2 minutes. Divide between two plates or bowls.
Garnish pasta with shredded mozzarella cheese and sliced green onion.
Serve warm.

NOTES

TREAT
YOURSELF
SIMPLE

A SIMPLE LIFE
IS A HAPPY LIFE

NOTES

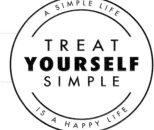

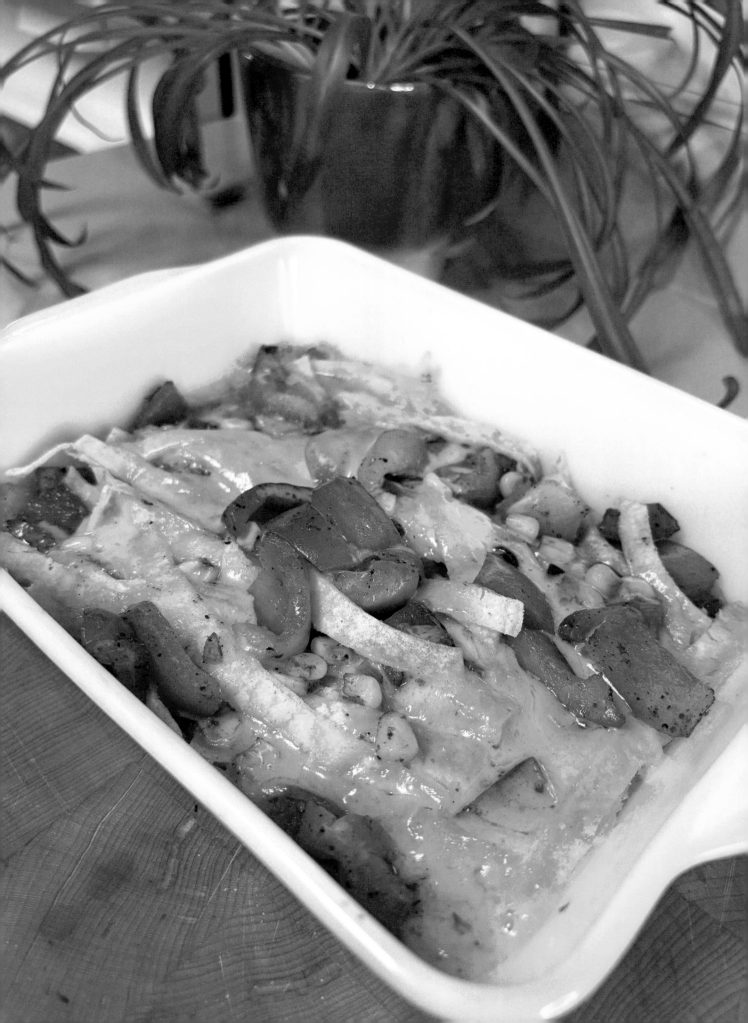

AUTUMN MEXICAN CASSEROLE OVEN

Serving Size:	2 servings	Cook time:	20 minutes
Prep time:	15 minutes	Needed:	Large skillet, loaf pan, heat-safe spoon

DIRECTIONS

○ Preheat oven to 400° F. Coat loaf pan with cooking spray. Set aside.

1 ➤ Bell Pepper, any color, chopped
¼ ➤ Peppers, Jalapeno, diced
2 T ➤ Onion, red, chopped
⅓ C ➤ Corn, fresh or frozen
¼ t ➤ Chili Powder
½ t ➤ Cumin, ground
dash ➤ Kosher Salt

○ Add olive oil to skillet over medium-high heat. Add above ingredients.
Sauté until browning on the outside of the peppers appears.
Remove and set aside.

¾ C ➤ Cheese, Mexican, shredded
4 ➤ Tortillas, Corn, cut into thin strips
½ can ➤ Refried Beans (mix with a little bit of water to make them easier to spread)
⅓ C ➤ Enchilada Sauce

○ Spread a little bit of enchilada sauce on the bottom of the pan.
Layer in order: half of the tortilla strips, ALL the beans, half of the veggies
mixture, half of the remaining enchilada sauce, half of the cheese.
Cover with the other half of the tortilla strips, veggies mixture,
enchilada sauce, and cheese.

○ Cover with foil. Bake for 15–20 minutes, until the sauce is bubbling
and the cheese is melted. Remove from heat. Divide into two servings.

➤ Cilantro, fresh
➤ Avocado slices
➤ Sour Cream

○ Top with guacamole, fresh cilantro, and sour cream.
Serve warm.

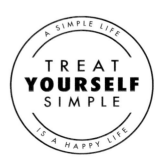

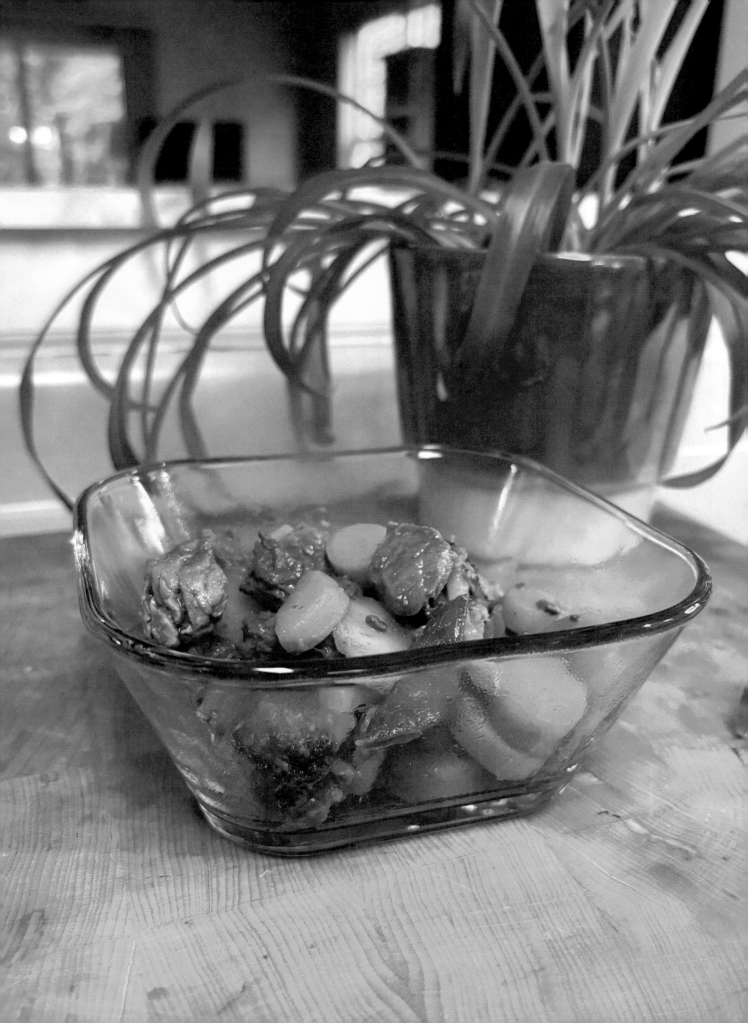

BEEF & VEGETABLE STIR-FRY STOVE

Serving Size:	2 servings	Cook time:	15 minutes
Prep time:	15 minutes	Needed:	Large skillet, heat-safe spoon

DIRECTIONS

1T ➤ Olive Oil

1 C ➤ Beef, roast, cut into bite-sized pieces

○ Coat skillet with olive oil over medium heat. Add beef; brown for 3-4 minutes, stirring and flipping occasionally.

1 pkg ➤ Vegetables, mixed, frozen, 10 oz, or use 2 C whatever fresh veggies you like.

○ Add above ingredient, stirring occasionally, cooking for 4-5 minutes.

1 t ➤ Flour

½ C ➤ Stir Fry Sauce

○ Add above ingredients to skillet. Stir to combine with vegetables.

○ Cover the skillet, cook over low heat for 5-8 minutes. Stir occasionally. Serve warm.

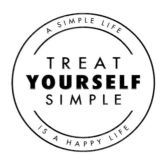

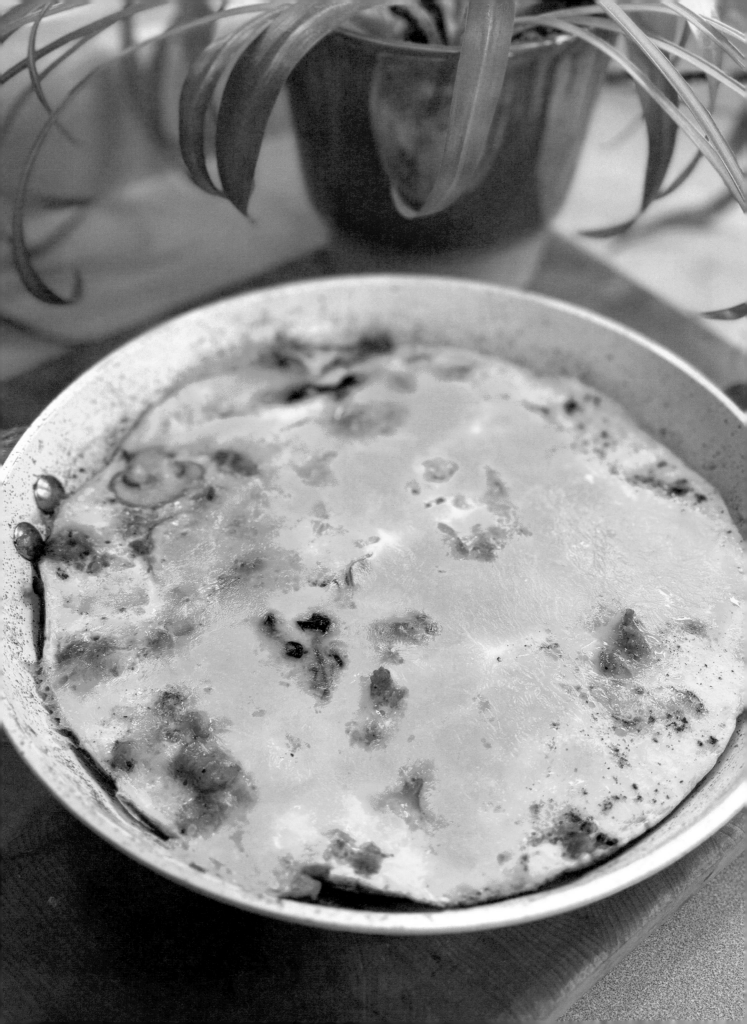

VEGGIE FR!TTATA WITH SAUSAGE 2/1 STOVE

Please note: Italian Sausage from Pasta with Pumpkin & Sausage 2/1

Serving Size:	2 servings	Cook time:	15 minutes
Prep time:	15 minutes	Needed:	Large skillet, measuring cup or small bowl, whisk, heat-safe spoon

DIRECTIONS

½ lb ➢ Sausage, ground, from **Pasta with Pumpkin & Sausage 2/1**
¾ C ➢ Spinach, baby, fresh
¼ C ➢ Bell Pepper, any color, chopped
¾ C ➢ Mushrooms, any type, fresh, sliced
¼ C ➢ Onion, sweet, fresh, chopped

○ Coat skillet with olive oil over medium heat. Add above ingredients to skillet; cook about 3–4 minutes until vegetables are tender, stirring occasionally.

4 ➢ Eggs, large, beaten
½ C ➢ Milk, any type
2 t ➢ Kosher Salt
dash ➢ Black Pepper, ground

○ Combine above ingredients in measuring cup or small bowl; whisk until blended. Pour egg mixture into skillet; cover; cook for 5–6 minutes until eggs are set.

½ C ➢ Cheese, Cheddar, shredded

○ Sprinkle cheese over egg mixture; turn heat off; cover for 2 minutes until cheese is melted. Divide between two plates. Serve warm.

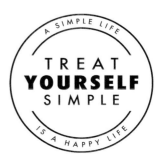

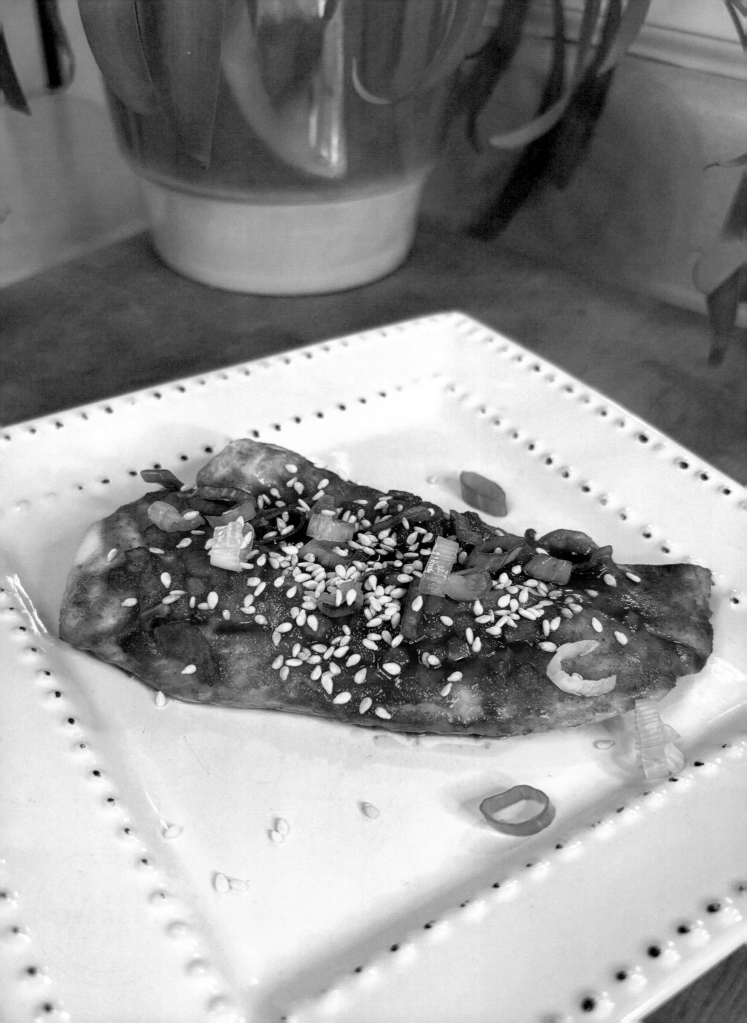

ASIAN SALMON GRILL OR OVEN

Serving Size:	2 servings	Cook time:	10 minutes
Prep time:	5 minutes	Needed:	Shallow bowl, baking sheet, spatula

DIRECTIONS

○ Preheat oven to 400º F or preheat grill to medium-high. Line baking sheet with aluminum foil. Set aside.

2 ➤ Salmon Filets, 4–6 oz each
1 t ➤ Ginger, fresh, peeled and grated or ¼ t ground ginger
1 t ➤ Garlic, minced
1 T ➤ Soy Sauce
2 T ➤ Worcestershire Sauce
2 T ➤ Sriracha Sauce

MARINADE

○ **Can make ahead. See Make Ahead Directions.** If not already prepared, add the above ingredients (besides the salmon) to a shallow dish.
Lastly coat salmon in mixture, coating evenly on each side.
Cover and marinate for 30 minutes or overnight.

○ Place salmon on a foil-lined baking sheet. Scrape all the excess marinade from the bowl onto the salmon.

GRILL

○ Slide foil packet from baking sheet onto grill; cook for 7–10 minutes.

OVEN

○ Bake for 10–12 minutes. With either option, salmon is done when top of salmon is caramelized and reaches 145º F.

½ t ➤ Sesame Seeds, toasted
1 ➤ Onion, green, chopped

○ Place one salmon filet on each of two plates.
Sprinkle above ingredients on salmon. Serve warm.

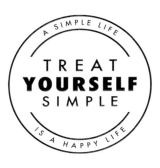

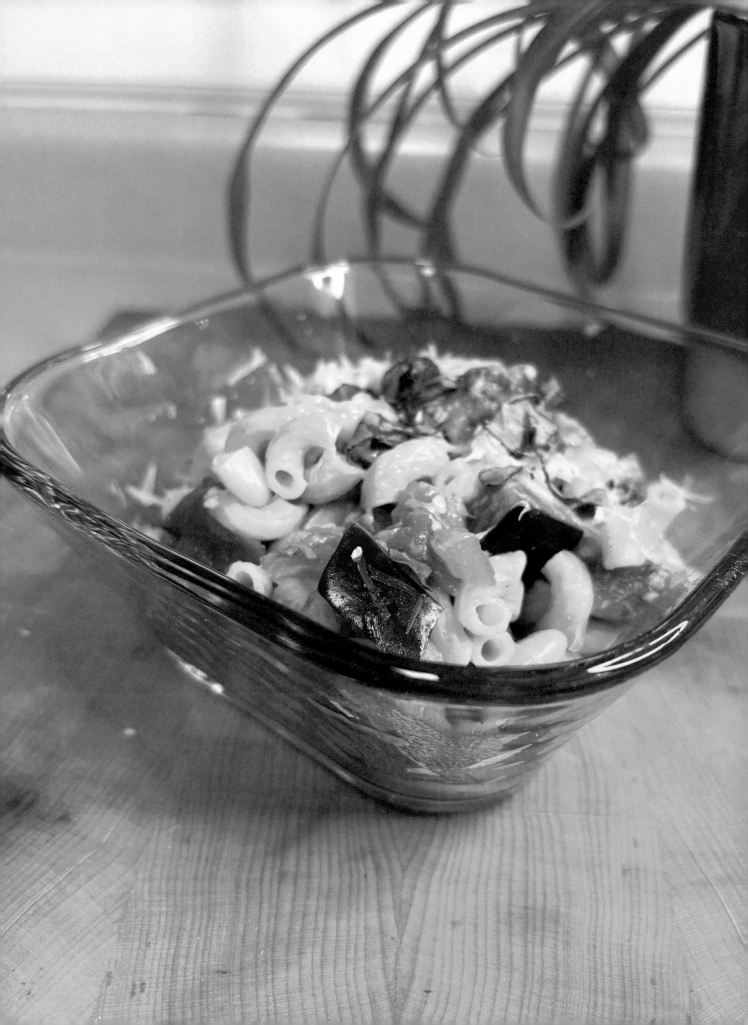

ONE-PAN HARVEST PASTA OVEN

Serving Size:	2 servings	Cook time:	20 minutes
Prep time:	20 minutes	Needed:	Large skillet, heat-safe spoon

DIRECTIONS

1 T ➤ Olive Oil
1 C ➤ Eggplant, small, fresh, cut into bite size pieces
¼ ➤ Zucchini, medium, fresh, chopped
1 ➤ Tomato, small, fresh, medium, chopped
1 T ➤ Onion, red, fresh, chopped
½ t ➤ Garlic, minced

○ Coat skillet with olive oil over medium heat. Add above ingredients to same skillet, stirring occasionally; cook uncovered for 7–10 minutes until the vegetables are almost tender,

¼ can ➤ Beans, cannellini, 15.5 oz can, rinsed and drained
½ C ➤ Broth, Chicken
½ C ➤ Pasta, elbow macaroni

○ Add the above ingredients to the skillet, bringing to a boil; reduce heat; cover and simmer for 7–10 minutes or until pasta is tender. Stir occasionally. Remove from heat.

dash ➤ Kosher Salt
dash ➤ Black Pepper, ground
optional ➤ Basil, fresh, chopped
optional ➤ Cheese, Parmesan, shredded

○ Divide pasta/vegetable mixture into two bowls. Sprinkle with salt & pepper. Top with basil and Parmesan cheese. Serve warm.

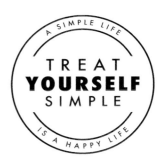

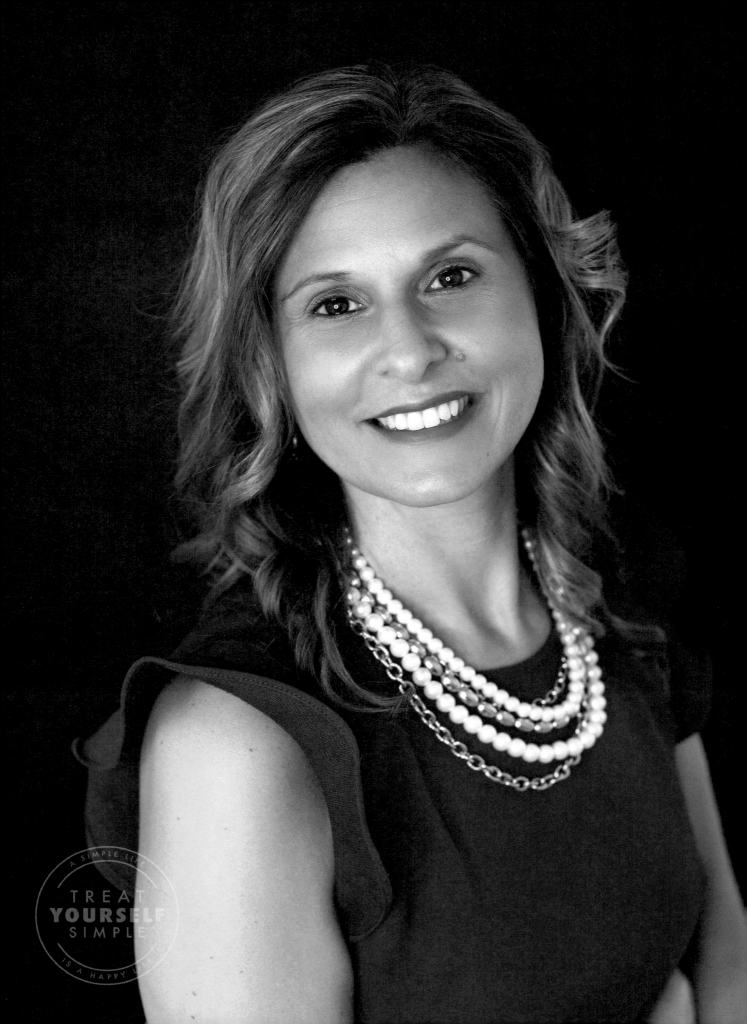

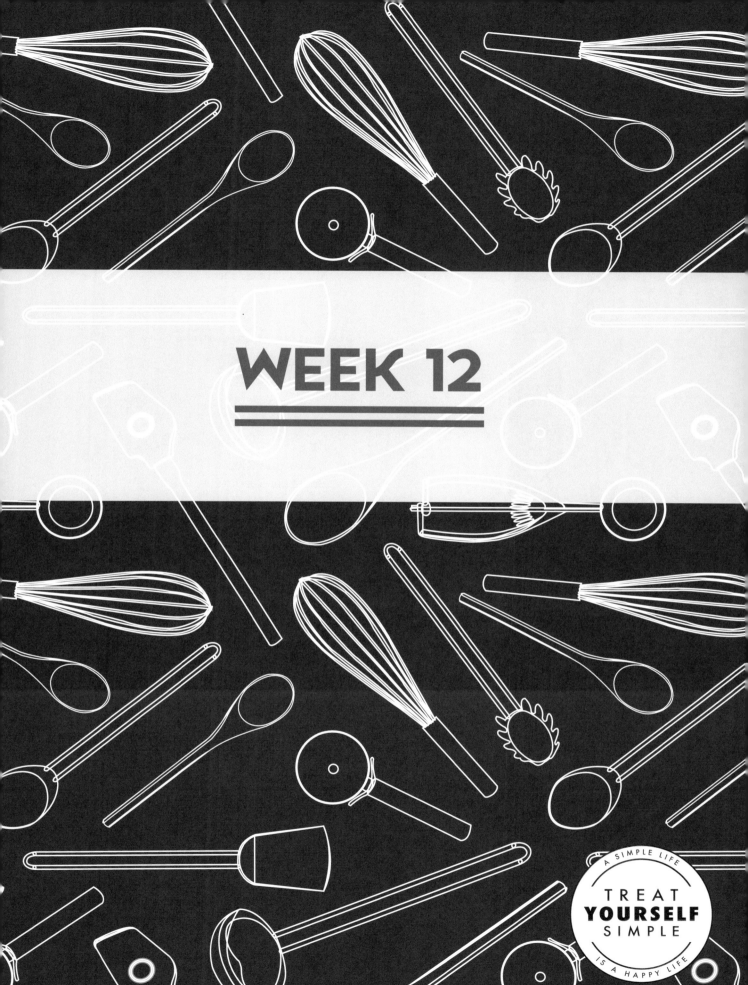

WEEK 12

WEEK 12 MENU PLAN

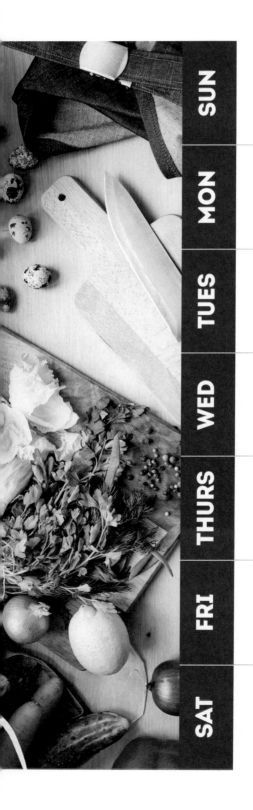

SUN

LIME PORK CHOPS

Green Beans
Multigrain Bread

MON

ASIAN TUNA NACHOS

Fresh Salad
Orange Slices

TUES

HONEY GARLIC CHICKEN 2/1

Jasmine Rice
Brussels Sprouts

WED

SPINACH, HAM & GRUYÈRE FRITTATA

Sweet Potato Discs
Cinnamon Apples

THURS

AUTUMN CRUNCH PASTA SALAD

Hummus
Celery Sticks

FRI

TEX MEX CHICKEN 2/1

Butternut Squash
Cinnamon Sliced Bananas

SAT

PINEAPPLE SHRIMP

Jasmine Rice
Fresh Green Beans

WEEK 12 GROCERY LIST

BY MEAL

LIME PORK CHOPS

2 T	Lime Juice
2 T	Soy Sauce
½ t	Maple Syrup
1½ t	Garlic, minced
1 T	Cilantro, fresh, chopped
2	Pork Chops, 4 oz each
dash	Kosher Salt
dash	Black Pepper, ground
½ T	Olive Oil

ASIAN TUNA NACHOS

1 T	Bell Pepper, any color, chopped
1 T	Celery, chopped
dash	Chili Powder
½ T	Cilantro, fresh, chopped
dash	Kosher Salt
1	Onion, green, chopped
½ T	Onion, red, chopped
1 T	Sesame Oil
1 T	Soy Sauce
1 can	Tuna, 5 oz, drained
½ C	Cheese, Cheddar, shredded
½ C	Avocado
½ C	Salsa
2 C	Tortilla Chips

HONEY GARLIC CHICKEN STIR FRY 2/1

⅓ C	Broth, Vegetable
1½ T	Honey
⅓ C	Soy Sauce
2 t	Flour
drizzle	Olive or Avocado Oil
4	Chicken Breasts, 4 oz each, cut into bite-sized pieces, half of chicken for **Tex Mex Chicken 2/1**
¼ C	Coconut Flakes

SPINACH, HAM & GRUYÈRE FRITTATA

4	Eggs, large
¼ t	Kosher Salt
¼ t	Black Pepper, ground
2 T	Milk
½ T	Olive Oil
1½ C	Spinach, baby, fresh
2 T	Garlic, minced
½ C	Ham, cooked, diced
2 T	Onion, sweet, chopped
½ T	Onion, green, fresh, chopped
4 T	Cheese, Gruyère shredded

AUTUMN CRUNCH PASTA SALAD

4 oz	Pasta, any type
2 oz	Spinach, baby, fresh
2 T	Apple Cider Vinegar
2 t	Cooking Wine
2 T	Honey
1 t	Paprika
1 t	Onion Powder
4 T	Olive Oil
1 t	Celery Seed
⅓ C	Celery, chopped
⅓ C	Cranberries, dried
½ can	Mandarin Oranges, 15 oz can, drained, or ¾ C
1	Apple, Granny Smith, thinly sliced
½ t	Lemon Juice
2 T	Walnuts, chopped
optional	Cheese, Feta

BY MEAL

TEX MEX CHICKEN 2/1

½ T	Olive Oil
½	Bell Pepper, any color, medium, sliced
1½ T	Garlic, minced
½ C	Onion, sweet, chopped
2	Chicken Breasts, cut into bite-sized pieces, 4 oz each, from **Honey Garlic Chicken 2/1**
½ t	Cumin, ground
½ t	Kosher Salt
dash	Black Pepper, ground
½ can	Beans, black, 15 oz can
½ can	Tomatoes, diced, 14 oz can
1½ t	Taco Seasoning
½ C	Corn, frozen
½ C	Cheese, Colby Jack, shredded
¼ C	Cilantro, fresh, chopped
¼ C	Onion, green, chopped
1	Zucchini, large, fresh, cut into bite-sized pieces

PINEAPPLE SHRIMP

1 T	Olive Oil
12	Shrimp, large, peeled and deveined, tail off or 2 C Salad Shrimp
½ t	Curry Powder
1 T	Soy Sauce
¼ t	Maple Syrup
1 T	Olive Oil
½	Bell Pepper, any color, chopped
¼ C	Carrots, fresh, shredded
1½ t	Garlic, minced
1 t	Ginger, fresh, peeled, grated
¼ C	Onion, fresh, sweet, chopped
½ can	Pineapple chunks, 14 oz can, drained, or ¾ C
3	Onions, green, fresh, chopped
¼ C	Peanuts, chopped
1	Lime, cut into wedges

WEEK 12 PREP

Cut 4 Chicken Breasts into bite-sized pieces ~ Honey Garlic Chicken 2/1, Tex Mex Chicken 2/1

Mince 19 Garlic cloves ~ Lime Pork Chops, Spinach Ham & Gruyère Frittata, Tex Mex Chicken 2/1, Pineapple Shrimp

Chop 1¼ Bell Pepper, any color ~ Asian Tuna Melt Nachos, Tex Mex Chicken 2/1, Pineapple Shrimp

Chop 2 stalks Celery ~ Asian Tuna Melt Nachos, Autumn Crunch Pasta Salad

Chop ⅛ Red Onion ~ Asian Tuna Melt Nachos

Chop 1¼ Sweet Onion ~ Spinach Ham & Gruyère Frittata; Tex Mex Chicken 2/1, Pineapple Shrimp

Chop 1 Zucchini into bite-sized pieces ~ Tex Mex Chicken 2/1

Shred 4 T Gruyère Cheese ~ Spinach Ham & Gruyère Frittata

Shred ½ C Colby Jack Cheese ~ Tex Mex Chicken 2/1

Shred ¼ C Carrot ~ Pineapple Shrimp

Chop 7 Green Onions ~ Asian Tuna Nachos, Spinach Ham & Gruyère Frittata, Tex Mex Chicken 2/1, Pineapple Shrimp

Shred ½ C Cheddar Cheese ~ Asian Tuna Nachos

Dice ½ C Ham ~ Spinach Ham & Gruyère Frittata

WEEK 12 MAKE AHEAD

Make Dressing ~ Autumn Crunch Pasta Salad

Taco Seasoning ~ Tex Mex Chicken 2/1

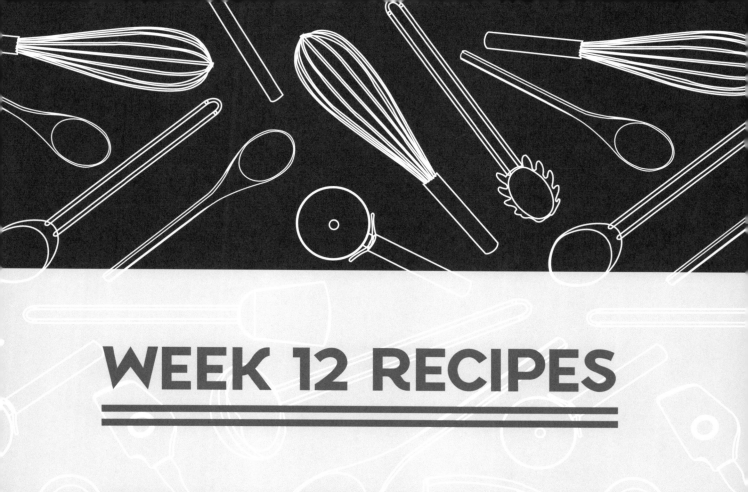

WEEK 12 RECIPES

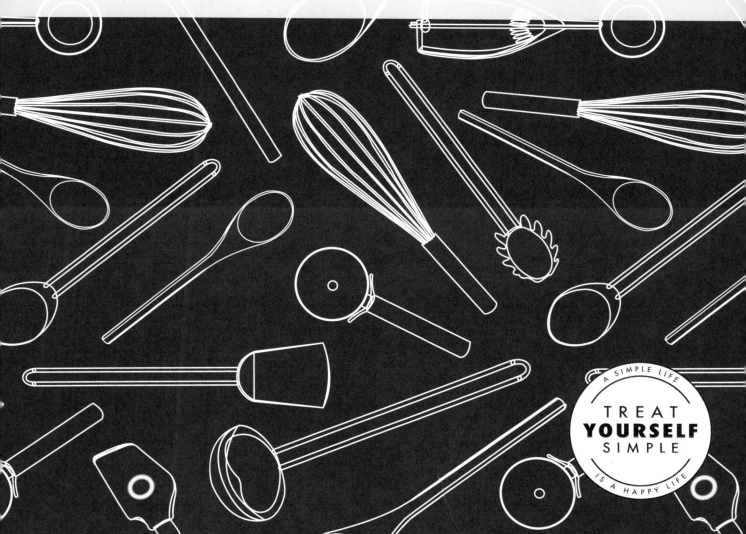

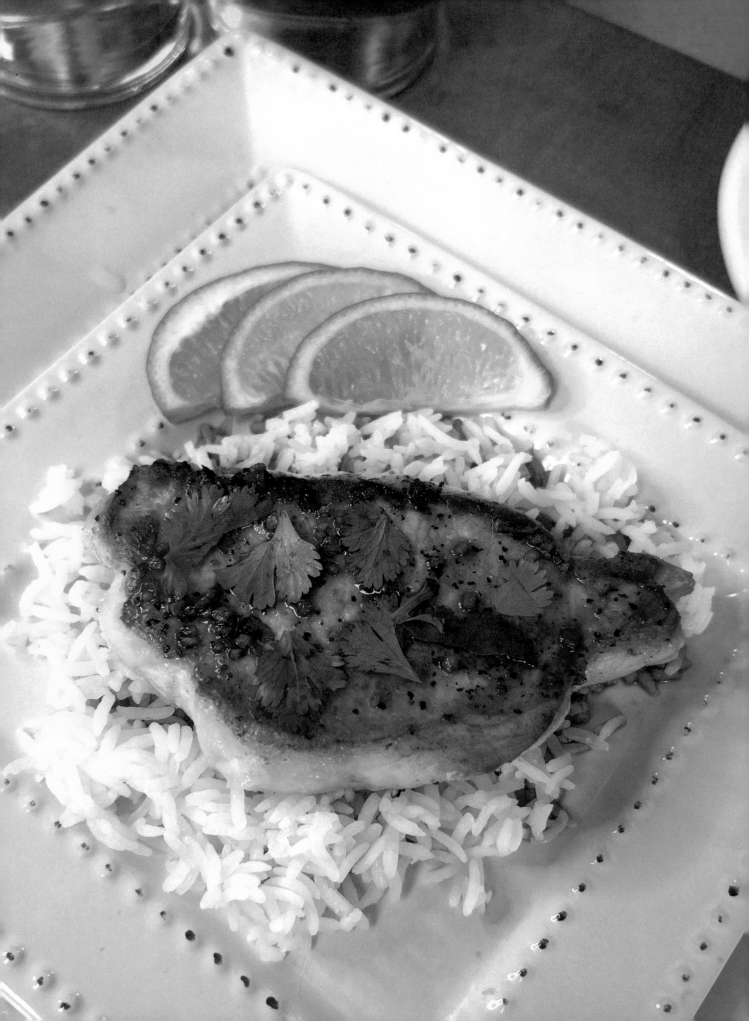

LIME PORK CHOPS GRILL OR STOVE

Serving Size:	2 servings	Cook time:	25 minutes
Prep time:	15 minutes	Needed:	Grill or skillet, small bowl, spatula, spoon

DIRECTIONS

2 T ⊳ Lime Juice
2 T ⊳ Soy Sauce
½ t ⊳ Maple Syrup
1½ t ⊳ Garlic, minced
1 T ⊳ Cilantro, fresh, chopped

○ In a small bowl, whisk together the ingredients listed above and 1 T of water. Set mixture aside.

2 ⊳ Pork Chops, 4 oz each
dash ⊳ Kosher Salt
dash ⊳ Black Pepper, ground
½ T ⊳ Olive Oil

○ Place pork chops on a plate and season generously on both sides with salt & pepper; then drizzle with oil and turn pork to coat.

GRILL

○ Heat grill to 350–400° F. Place on grill and cook each side for 5–6 minutes until done, internal temperature is 145° F. Place each pork chop on a plate. Spoon prepared sauce over pork chops. Serve warm.

STOVE

○ Heat skillet to medium-high. Place pork chops in skillet; cook on each side for 5–6 minutes until done. Place each pork chop on a plate. Spoon prepared sauce over pork chops. Serve warm.

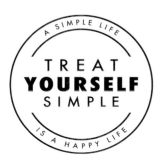

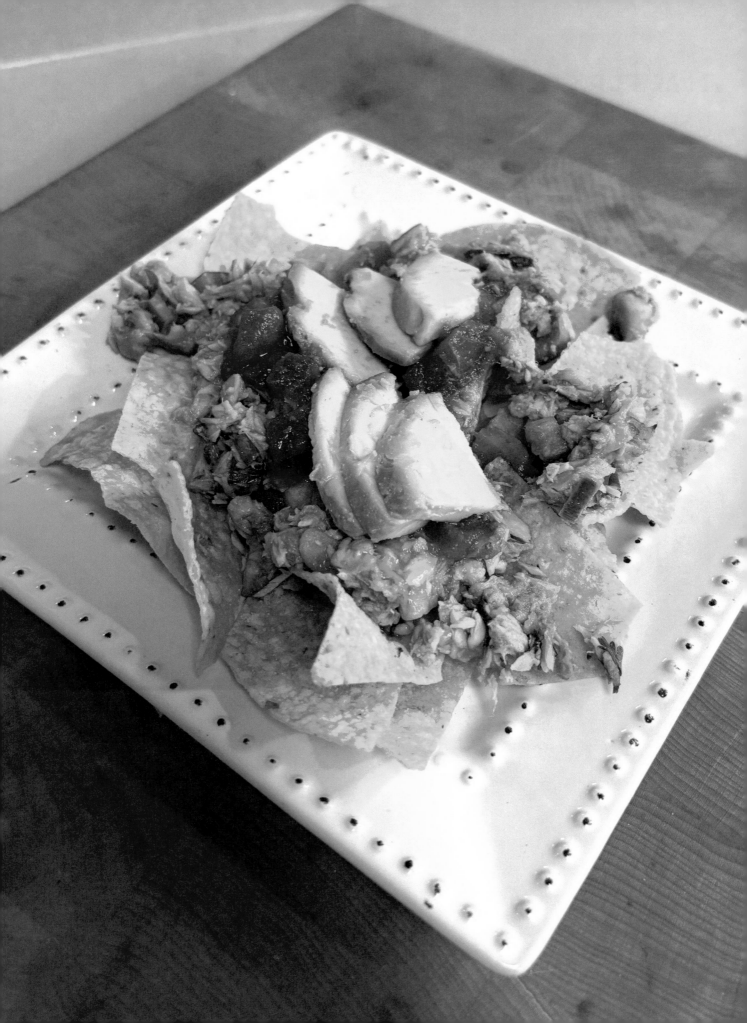

ASIAN TUNA NACHOS OVEN

Serving Size:	2 servings	Cook time:	5 minutes
Prep time:	15 minutes	Needed:	Baking sheet, medium bowl, spoon

DIRECTIONS

○ Preheat oven to 375º F. Line a baking sheet with aluminum foil; coat with cooking spray; set aside.

1 T ➤ Bell Pepper, any color, chopped
1 T ➤ Celery, chopped
dash ➤ Chili Powder
½ T ➤ Cilantro, fresh, chopped
dash ➤ Kosher Salt
1 ➤ Onion, green, chopped
½ T ➤ Onion, red, chopped
1 T ➤ Sesame Oil
1 T ➤ Soy Sauce
1 can ➤ Tuna, 5 oz can, drained

○ Combine the ingredients listed above in medium mixing bowl. Set aside.

½ C ➤ Cheese, Cheddar, shredded

○ On prepared baking sheet, place tuna mixture and sprinkle with cheese. Bake for 4–5 minutes, or until cheese is bubbly. Remove baking sheet from heat.

2 C ➤ Tortilla Chips
½ C ➤ Avocado
½ C ➤ Salsa

○ Divide chips onto two plates. Spread the tuna mixture on chips. Top with guacamole and salsa. Serve warm.

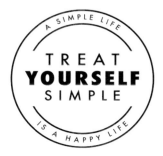

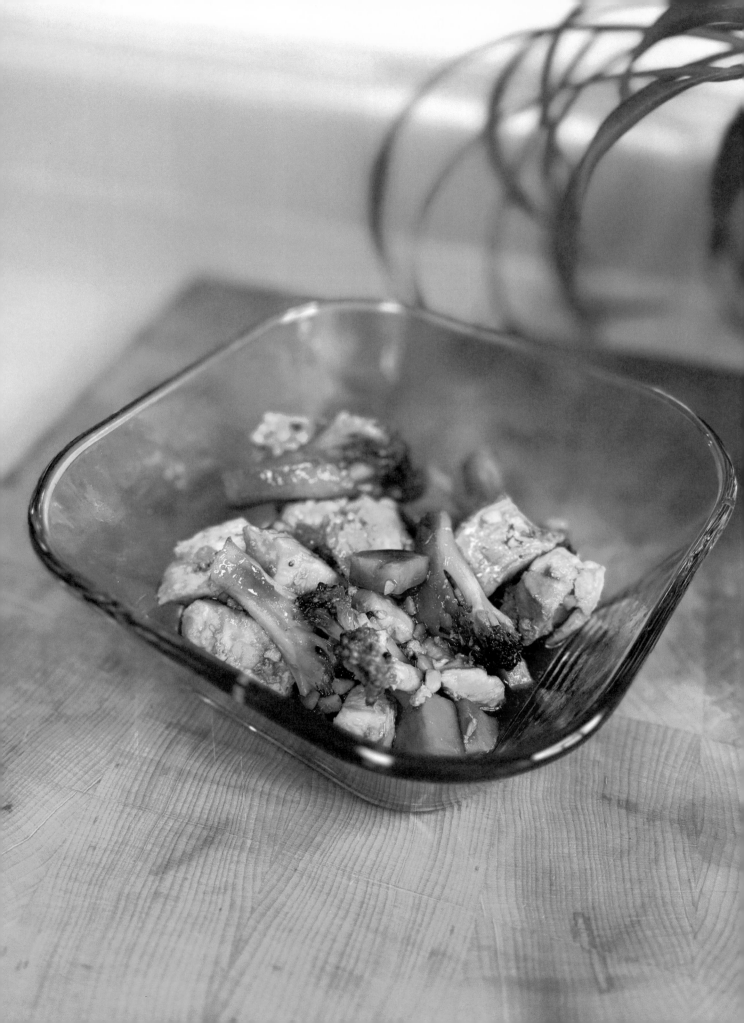

HONEY GARLIC CHICKEN 2/1 STOVE

Please note: Makes Chicken for Tex Mex Chicken 2/1

Serving Size:	2 servings	Cook time:	15 minutes
Prep time:	10 minutes	Needed:	Large skillet, measuring cup or small bowl, spatula

DIRECTIONS

⅓ C ➤ Broth, Vegetable
1½ T ➤ Honey
⅓ C ➤ Soy Sauce
2 t ➤ Flour

○ Whisk together broth, honey, soy sauce in measuring cup or small bowl. Add flour a little at a time, to thicken sauce. Set aside.

drizzle ➤ Olive or Avocado Oil
4 ➤ Chicken Breasts, 4 oz each, cut into bite-sized pieces

○ Coat skillet with olive oil over medium heat. Once heated, add chicken. Cook for 2–5 minutes until pink begins to disappear. Don't forget to stir occasionally.

NOTE: *Remove half of the chicken for* **Tex Mex Chicken 2/1.** *Set aside, cool, and store in an airtight container. Refrigerate for 7–10 days.*

○ Add sauce to skillet. Cook an addiditonal 3–4 minutes.

¼ C ➤ Coconut Flakes

○ Divide into two servings. Sprinkle coconut flakes. Serve warm.

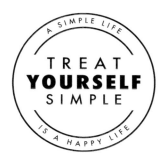

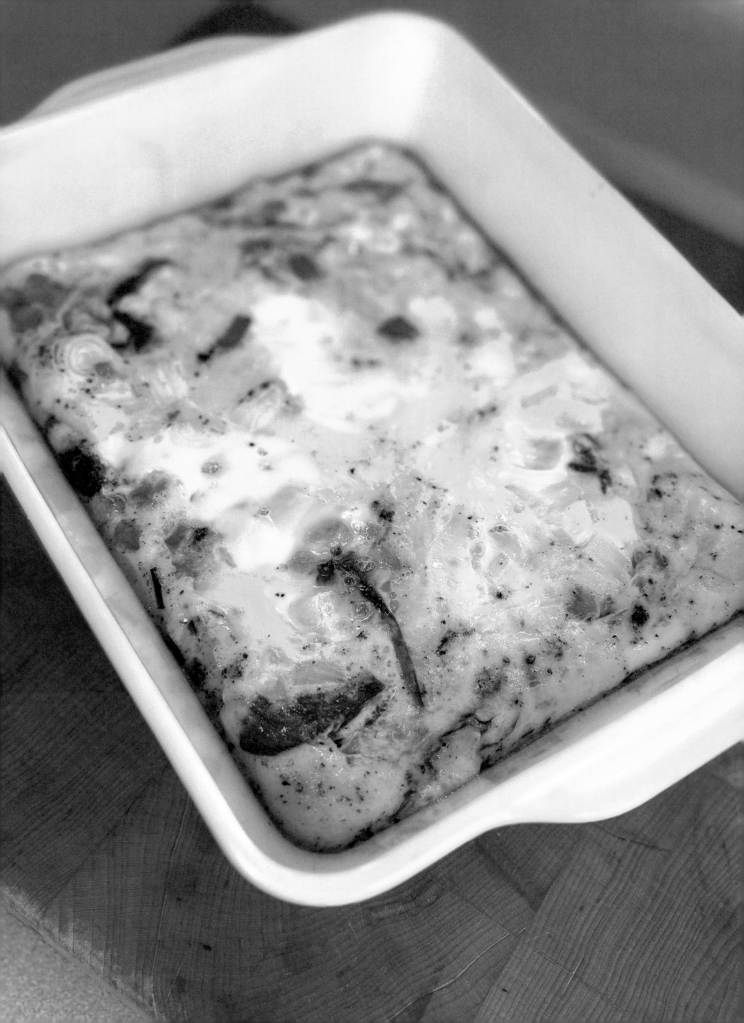

SPINACH, HAM & GRUYÈRE FRITTATA   OVEN

Serving Size:	2 servings	Cook time:	30 minutes
Prep time:	15 minutes	Needed:	Large skillet, casserole dish, measuring cup or small bowl, whisk, heat-safe spoon

DIRECTIONS

○ Preheat oven to 375° F. Coat a casserole dish with cooking spray. Set aside.

4 ➤ Eggs, large
¼ t ➤ Kosher Salt
¼ t ➤ Black Pepper, ground
2 T ➤ Milk

○ Combine above ingredients in measuring cup or small bowl; whisk together. Set aside.

½ T ➤ Olive Oil
1½ C ➤ Spinach, baby, fresh
2 T ➤ Garlic, minced

○ Heat oil in large skillet over medium heat. Add above ingredients; sauté for 3–5 minutes until tender. Place in prepared casserole dish.

½ C ➤ Ham, cooked, diced
2 T ➤ Onion, sweet, chopped
½ T ➤ Onions, green, fresh, chopped
4 T ➤ Cheese, Gruyère, shredded

○ Layer ham, onion, and chives in the same casserole dish. Sprinkle with cheese. Pour the egg mixture over top of cheese. Cook in oven for 20–25 minutes or until toothpick comes out clean. Divide into two servings. Serve warm.

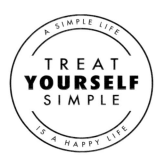

A SIMPLE LIFE
TREAT
YOURSELF
SIMPLE
IS A HAPPY LIFE

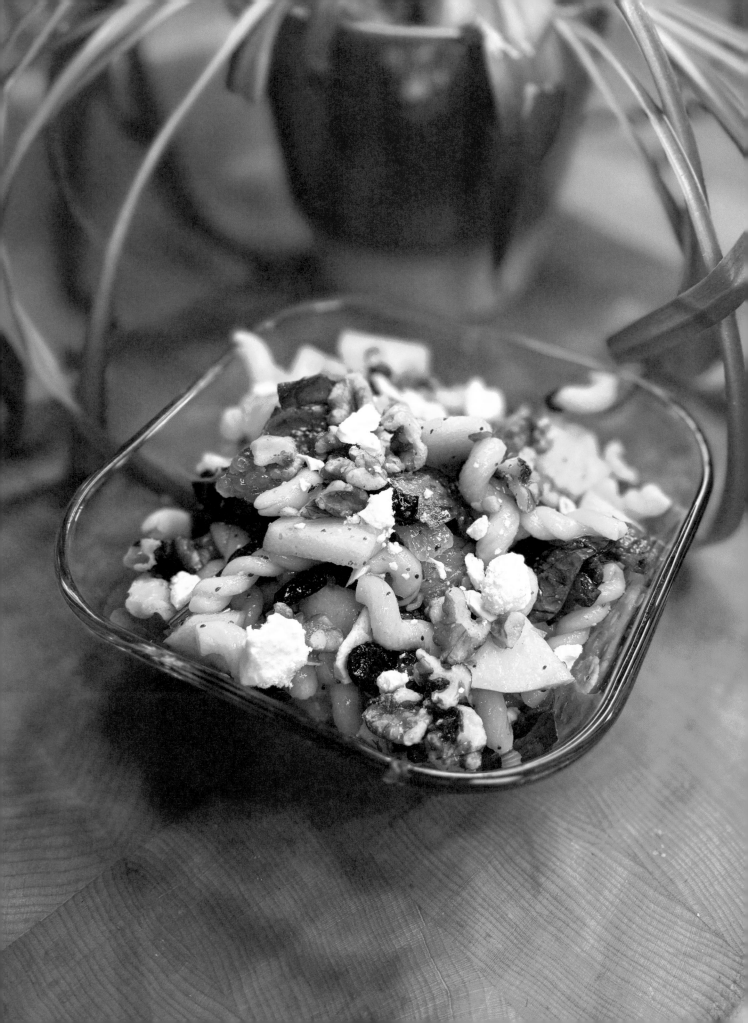

AUTUMN CRUNCH PASTA SALAD STOVE

Serving Size:	2 servings	Cook time:	15 minutes
Prep time:	20 minutes	Needed:	Medium saucepan, medium bowl, heat-safe spoon

DIRECTIONS

4oz ➢ Pasta, any type

○ Cook pasta according to package directions; drain and place in medium bowl.

2 oz ➢ Spinach, baby, fresh

○ Add spinach to pasta in bowl; stir to combine. Spinach will begin to wilt a little. Chill in refrigerator for 10–15 minutes or until desired coolness is reached.

2 T ➢ Apple Cider Vinegar
2 t ➢ Cooking Wine
2 T ➢ Honey
1 t ➢ Paprika
1 t ➢ Onion Powder
4 T ➢ Olive Oil
1 t ➢ Celery Seed

DRESSING

○ **Can make ahead. See Make Ahead Directions.** If not already prepared, combine the above ingredients in a jar with a tight-fitting lid.
Shake the dressing until smooth and season with salt & pepper to taste.
Set in fridge until ready to use.

⅓ C ➢ Celery, chopped
⅓ C ➢ Cranberries, dried
½ can ➢ Mandarin Oranges, drained, 15 oz can, drained, or ¾ C
1 ➢ Apple, Granny Smith, thinly sliced
½ t ➢ Lemon Juice

○ Remove bowl with pasta/spinach mixture from refrigerator. Add celery, dried cranberries, apples and mandarin oranges into bowl.
Pour dressing over salad mixture and toss to combine.

2 T ➢ Walnuts, chopped
optional ➢ Cheese, Feta

○ Divide salad/pasta mixture between two plates or bowls.
Top with walnuts and feta cheese. Serve immediately.

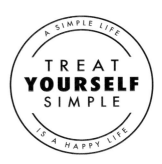

A SIMPLE LIFE
TREAT
YOURSELF
SIMPLE
IS A HAPPY LIFE

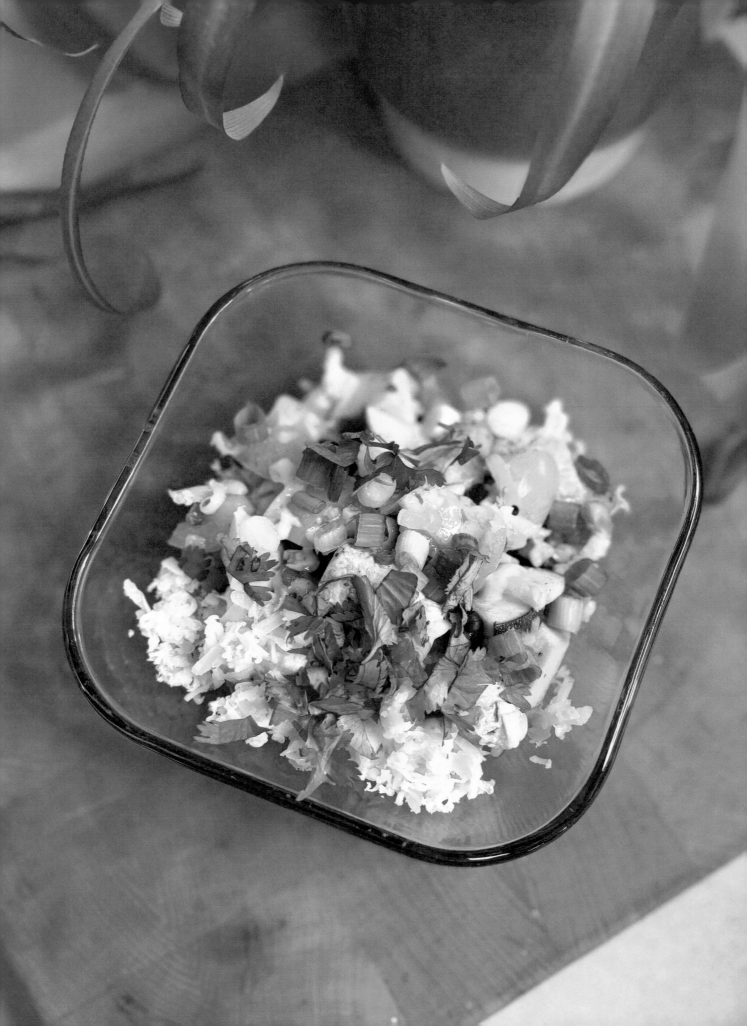

TEX MEX CHICKEN 2/1 STOVE

Please note: Chicken was prepared from Honey Garlic Chicken 2/1

Serving Size:	2 servings	Cook time:	20 minutes
Prep time:	10 minutes	Needed:	Large skillet, heat-safe spoon

DIRECTIONS

½ T ➤ Olive Oil
½ ➤ Bell Pepper, any color, medium, sliced
1½ T ➤ Garlic, minced
½ C ➤ Onion, sweet, chopped

○ Coat skillet with olive oil over medium-low heat. Add the above ingredients; cook for 3 minutes stirring occasionally. Move mixture to side of skillet.

2 ➤ Chicken Breasts, 4 oz each from **Honey Garlic Chicken 2/1,** cut into bite-sized pieces
½ t ➤ Cumin, ground
½ t ➤ Kosher Salt
dash ➤ Black Pepper, ground

○ Add the chicken to other side of the skillet; sprinkle with the above seasonings; cook for about 5 minutes stirring occasionally.

○ Stir together pepper mixture and cooked chicken.

½ can ➤ Beans, black, 15 oz can
½ can ➤ Tomatoes, diced, 14 oz can
1½ t ➤ Taco Seasoning
½ C ➤ Corn, frozen
1 ➤ Zucchini, large, fresh, cut into bite-sized pieces

○ Add the above ingredients to skillet; stir, cover, and cook on medium-low for 10 minutes.

½ C ➤ Cheese, Colby Jack, shredded
¼ C ➤ Cilantro, fresh, chopped
¼ C ➤ Onion, green, chopped

○ Sprinkle mixture with cheese, cover and cook for 2–3 minutes or until cheese has melted. Divide between two plates. Top with green onion and cilantro. Serve warm.

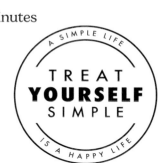

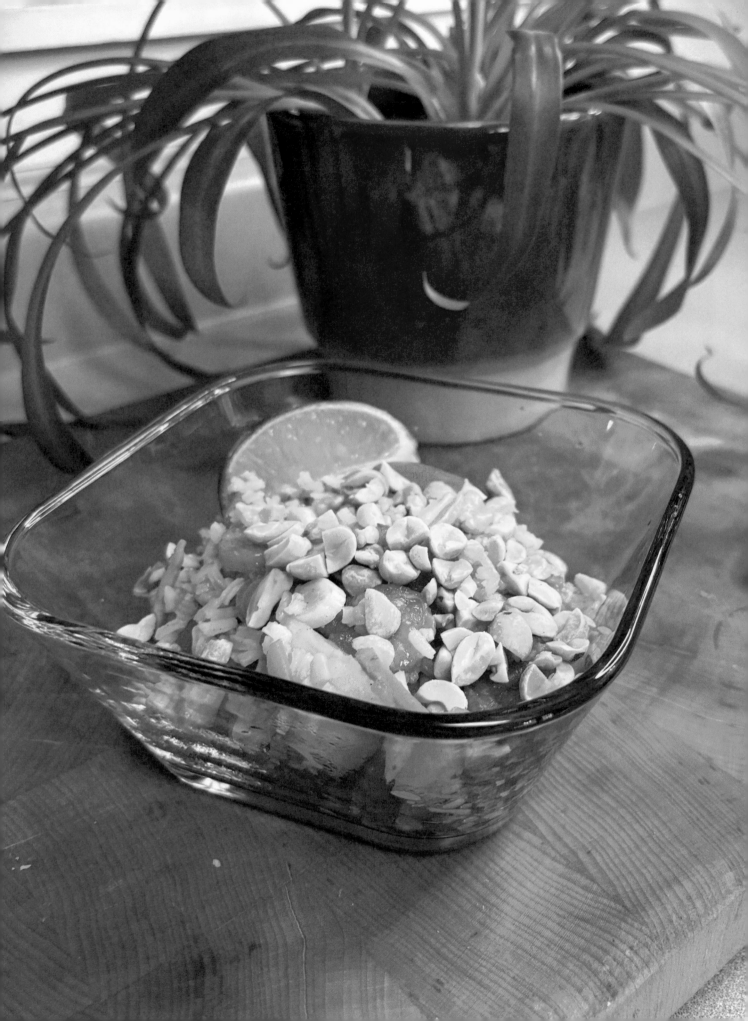

PINEAPPLE SHRIMP STOVE

Serving Size:	2 servings	Cook time:	20 minutes
Prep time:	15 minutes	Needed:	Small mixing bowl, large skillet, heat-safe spoon

DIRECTIONS

1 T ➤ Olive Oil
12 ➤ Shrimp, large, peeled and deveined, tail off or 2 C Salad Shrimp
½ t ➤ Curry Powder
1 T ➤ Soy Sauce
¼ t ➤ Maple Syrup

○ Coat skillet with olive oil over medium-high heat. Add above ingredients. Stir frequently for 2–3 minutes or until shrimp turns pink; remove from skillet. Set aside.

1 T ➤ Olive Oil
½ ➤ Bell Pepper, any color, chopped
¼ C ➤ Carrots, fresh, shredded
¼ C ➤ Onion, sweet, chopped
1½ t ➤ Garlic, minced
1 t ➤ Ginger, fresh, peeled, grated

○ Coat skillet with olive oil over medium-high heat. Add above ingredients; stir frequently for 4 minutes.

½ can ➤ Pineapple, chunks, 14 oz can, drained, or ¾ C

○ Add pineapple and prepared shrimp to same skillet; stir together. Heat through over medium heat until desired temperature is reached. Remove from heat..

3 ➤ Onions, green, fresh, chopped
¼ C ➤ Peanuts, chopped
1 ➤ Lime, cut into wedges

○ Stir in green onions. Divide between two plates or bowls. Sprinkle with peanuts. Squeeze lime wedges over the top of mixture and drizzle juice for more flavor. Serve warm.

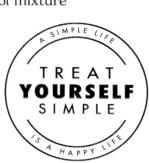

INDEX

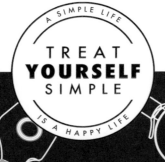

SEAFOOD

EGGS

VEGETABLE-BASED

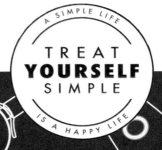

A SIMPLE LIFE

TREAT
YOURSELF
SIMPLE

IS A HAPPY LIFE

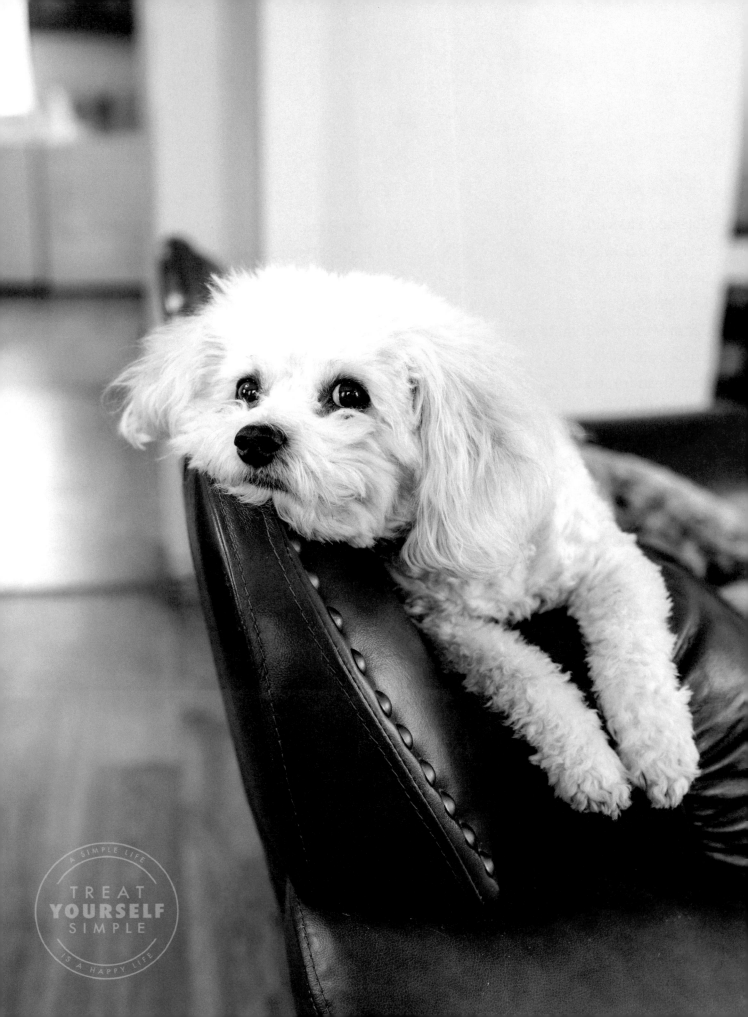